Physician's Guide to Non-Insulin-Dependent (Type II) Diabetes: Diagnosis and Treatment

American Diabetes Association, Inc., Alexandria, Virginia 22314
© 1984, 1988 by the American Diabetes Association, Inc. All rights reserved
First edition published 1984. Second edition 1988
First printing March 1984. Second printing October 1984. Third printing 1988
Printed in the United States of America
ISBN 0-945448-00-7

Contents

Introduction

Since the first appearance of the *Physician's Guide* in 1984, it has become a key reference handbook for all health-care professionals involved in the care and treatment of people with non-insulin-dependent (type II) diabetes mellitus. The second edition of the *Guide* is presented in the same easy-to-use format as the original, and sections have been updated and expanded with newly available information.

The major revisions in this edition are the sections on pathogenesis, management, and detection and treatment of complications. The editorial board carefully reviewed recent literature that supports the changes made, and the consultant reviewers agreed with the revisions. It is becoming clear that blood glucose regulation and attention to blood pressure and proper diet are key elements in the management of type II diabetes. Nevertheless, the complications of diabetes are still troublesome and demand early detection and treatment to control the potentially devastating impact of this disease.

The second edition of the *Guide* is part of ADA's growing Clinical Education Program (CEP) library, which also currently includes the *Physician's Guide to Insulin-Dependent (Type I) Diabetes Mellitus: Diagnosis and Treatment; Goals for Diabetes Education;* and *Clinical Diabetes Reviews, Volume 1.* The CEP library is being developed to provide the primary-care physician with both the basic and comprehensive information needed to treat patients with diabetes mellitus.

ADA hopes that you will find the second edition of the *Guide* as useful as the first and that it will encourage you to add other ADA publications to your library that can help you manage your patients with diabetes mellitus more effectively.

JOHN A. COLWELL, MD, PhD
President, American Diabetes Association

A Word About This Guide

The *Physician's Guide* was originally developed in 1984 to provide the primary-care physician with a single, practical reference on the diagnosis and management of non-insulin-dependent diabetes mellitus (type II diabetes mellitus or NIDDM). The objective of the *Guide* was to help the practitioner provide the best possible medical care to patients with this type of diabetes.

The way in which the original *Guide* was developed may give the practitioner an appreciation of its value. First, nine contributing editors—a cross section of the most renowned research and clinical specialists in diabetes mellitus—compiled the latest information on pathogenesis, diagnosis, and treatment of type II diabetes, emphasizing the specific clinical applications of this information. The manuscript was then reviewed, debated, and improved at a meeting of the contributors together with seven additional specialists in diabetes. These 16 authorities reached a consensus on guidelines for diagnosis and treatment—a consensus solidly rooted in the body of knowledge in this field at that time.

The manuscript was then evaluated by a panel of consultants in other specialties. These consultants were designated by eight medical societies whose members in one way or another treat patients with diabetes and can therefore be expected to be users of the *Guide*. The societies were

- American Academy of Family Physicians (AAFP)
- American Academy of Ophthalmology (AAO)
- American College of Physicians (ACP)
- American Geriatrics Society (AGS)
- American Medical Association (AMA)
- American Osteopathic Association (AOA)
- American Society of Internal Medicine (ASIM)
- National Medical Association (NMA)

All the contributors and consultants are listed on pages xiii–xvi.

In addition to the careful attention that went into the preparation of the contents, considerable effort was made to ensure that the *Guide* would be practical and useful. It was designed to help the practitioner resolve problems and concerns.

To gain familiarity with the *Guide*, I suggest you do the following before you begin to read it:

Note that we have listed not only the five main chapters, which are tabbed for easy access, but also the major sections within each chapter. Also note that the section headings are recapitulated on the tabbed dividers.

2. Read the "Highlights" at the beginning of each chapter. The highlights are summaries that capture the essential information presented in the *Guide*.

It is apparent that there are unanswered questions concerning diagnosis and treatment of type II diabetes mellitus. However, the knowledge at hand, although far from complete, is sufficient to encourage efforts to improve the management of patients with type II diabetes. It is to help attain this objective that the American Diabetes Association has published the *Guide*.

We hope the *Guide* will occupy a space on your bookshelf along with your most trusted and well-thumbed reference books.

HAROLD RIFKIN, MD
Editor-in-Chief

About the Second Edition . . .

Advances in understanding the pathophysiology of type II diabetes mellitus and its complications are leading to dramatic changes in the treatment of this disorder. Because the purpose of the *Physician's Guide to Non-Insulin-Dependent (Type II) Diabetes: Diagnosis and Treatment* is to provide the primary-care physician with a source of information to help provide the best possible medical care to patients with type II diabetes, it is essential that the *Guide* be updated on a regular basis. This ensures that the rapid advances being made in clinical investigation are translated into improved care for the patient with type II diabetes.

The major revisions in this edition of the *Guide* are found in the sections on pathogenesis, management, and detection and treatment of complications. Much new information supports the important roles of blood glucose regulation, blood pressure control, and blood lipid and lipoprotein normalization as key features in preventing or modifying the chronic complications of diabetic mellitus. More aggressive detection of early microvascular and macrovascular complications is now important because appropriate early therapeutic interventions have been shown to be beneficial in lessening the sequelae of these complications.

The members of the committee who participated in making this revision strove to maintain the high quality and useful practical approach that has made the *Guide* so helpful to the primary-care physician who takes care of patients with type II diabetes.

HAROLD LEBOVITZ, MD
Editor, Second Edition

Contributors of the
Second Edition

Editor-in-Chief   **HAROLD E. LEBOVITZ, MD**
State University of New York
  Health Science Center
Brooklyn, New York

Contributing
Editors

CHARLES M. CLARK, JR., MD
Indiana University School of Medicine
Indianapolis, Indiana

RALPH A. DeFRONZO, MD
Yale University School of Medicine
New Haven, Connecticut

JACK GERICH, MD
University of Pittsburgh
Pittsburgh, Pennsylvania

ROBERT KREISBERG, MD
University of Alabama School of Medicine
Birmingham, Alabama

DEAN LOCKWOOD, MD
University of Rochester School of Medicine
Rochester, New York

ARLAN ROSENBLOOM, MD
University of Florida School of Medicine
Gainesville, Florida

JAY S. SKYLER, MD
University of Miami School of Medicine
Miami, Florida

FRANK VINICOR, MD
Indiana University School of Medicine
Indianapolis, Indiana

BRUCE ZIMMERMAN, MD
Mayo Clinic
Rochester, Minnesota

Diabetes
Consultants

STEFAN FAJANS, MD
University of Michigan School of Medicine
Ann Arbor, Michigan

SHERMAN M. HOLVEY, MD
UCLA School of Medicine
Los Angeles, California

EDWARD S. HORTON, MD
University of Vermont College of Medicine
Burlington, Vermont

HAROLD RIFKIN, MD
Albert Einstein College of Medicine
New York, New York

JOHN RUNYAN, JR., MD
University of Tennessee School of Medicine
Memphis Tennessee

FRED WHITEHOUSE, MD
Henry Ford Hospital
Detroit, Michigan

Contributors of the First Edition

Editor-in-Chief   HAROLD RIFKIN, MD
Albert Einstein College of Medicine
New York, New York

Contributing   GEORGE F. CAHILL, JR., MD
Editors   Howard Hughes Medical Institute
Bethesda, Maryland

JOHN A. COLWELL, MD, PhD
Charleston VA Medical Center
Charleston, South Carolina

RALPH A. DeFRONZO, MD
Yale University School of Medicine
New Haven, Connecticut

SHERMAN M. HOLVEY, MD
UCLA School of Medicine
Los Angeles, California

EDWARD S. HORTON, MD
University of Vermont College of Medicine
Burlington, Vermont

HAROLD E. LEBOVITZ, MD
State University of New York
    Health Science Center
Brooklyn, New York

JERROLD M. OLEFSKY, MD
University of California, San Diego,
    School of Medicine
San Diego, California

JAY S. SKYLER, MD
University of Miami School of Medicine
Miami, Florida

Diabetes   RONALD A. ARKY, MD
Consultants   Harvard Medical School at Mount Auburn Hospital
Cambridge, Massachusetts

CHARLES M. CLARK, JR., MD
Indiana University School of Medicine
Indianapolis, Indiana

ALLAN L. DRASH, MD
Children's Hospital of Pittsburgh
Pittsburgh, Pennsylvania

SAUL M. GENUTH, MD
Case Western Reserve University School of Medicine
Cleveland, Ohio

DOROTHY GOHDES, MD
Indian Health Service Diabetes Program
Albuquerque, New Mexico

PHILIP RASKIN, MD
University of Texas Health Science Center at Dallas
Dallas, Texas

KARL E. SUSSMAN, MD
Denver VA Medical Center
Denver, Colorado

Consultants
in Other
Specialties

WALTER M. BORTZ II, MD
American Geriatrics Society

JOHN H. BURNETT, DO
American Osteopathic Association

JACK M. COLWILL, MD
Society of Teachers of Family Medicine

MATTHEW D. DAVIS, MD
American Academy of Ophthalmology

HAROLD HIGH, MD
American Academy of Family Physicians

A. HAROLD LUBIN, MD
American Medical Association

MURRAY PIZETTE, MD
American College of Physicians

C. BURNS ROEHRIG, MD
American Society of Internal Medicine

JOHN TOWNSEND, MD
National Medical Association

Endorsing Organizations of the First Edition

The *Physician's Guide* has been endorsed by the following medical societies:

American Academy of Family Physicians
American Academy of Ophthalmology
American Geriatrics Society
American Medical Association
American Society of Internal Medicine

Diagnosis and Classification of Diabetes Mellitus

Highlights

Diabetes mellitus (DM) is a disorder characterized by fasting hyperglycemia or plasma glucose levels above defined limits during oral glucose tolerance testing. There are three clinical subclasses of diabetes mellitus:

Insulin-dependent diabetes mellitus (type I or IDDM): approximately 10 percent of known cases of diabetes in the United States are type I.

Non-insulin-dependent diabetes mellitus (type II or NIDDM): approximately 90 percent of all known cases of diabetes in the United States are type II.

Other types: patients with other types of diabetes mellitus have known or very likely causes for diabetes.

Patients with impaired glucose tolerance (IGT) have plasma glucose levels that are higher than normal but not diagnostic for diabetes mellitus. About 25 percent of patients with IGT eventually develop diabetes mellitus.

Patients with gestational diabetes mellitus (GDM) have onset or discovery of glucose intolerance during pregnancy, usually in the second or third trimester.

Distinguishing characteristics of these categories of glucose intolerance are summarized in Table 1, page 4.

Candidates for screening tests include
- people with a strong family history of diabetes mellitus,
- people who are markedly obese,
- women with a morbid obstetrical history or a history of babies over 9 pounds at birth,
- all pregnant women between 24 and 28 weeks of pregnancy, and
- individuals with recurrent skin, genital, or urinary tract infections.

Criteria for positive screening tests are summarized in Table 4, page 8.

Indications for diagnostic testing include
- positive screening test results,
- obvious signs and symptoms of diabetes mellitus (polydipsia, polyuria, polyphagia, weight loss), and
- an incomplete clinical picture, such as glucosuria or equivocal elevation of random plasma glucose level.

Criteria for diagnosis of diabetes mellitus, impaired glucose tolerance, and gestational diabetes are summarized in Table 5, page 10.

Before treatment, a complete evaluation should be made to determine
- the type of diabetes or glucose intolerance,
- the presence of underlying diseases that need further evaluation, and
- the presence of complications.

Diagnosis and Classification of Diabetes Mellitus

INTRODUCTION

Diabetes mellitus is a chronic disorder characterized by abnormalities in the metabolism of carbohydrate, protein, and fat; it is often accompanied, after some time, by specific microvascular, macrovascular, and neuropathic complications.

It is now recognized that diabetes mellitus encompasses a group of genetically and clinically heterogeneous disorders in which glucose intolerance is a common denominator. Thus, although diabetes mellitus affects the metabolism of all body fuels, its diagnosis depends on identification of specific plasma glucose abnormalities.

Because the syndrome of diabetes mellitus encompasses many disorders that differ in pathogenesis, natural history, and responses to treatment, it is important that clinicians and researchers use commonly accepted terminology as well as standardized classification and diagnostic criteria when categorizing patients with glucose intolerance.

In the past, uniform criteria were lacking for the diagnosis of diabetes mellitus and the classification of its various types. Consistency of nomenclature for this heterogeneous disorder was sought for a variety of reasons: to perform valid epidemiologic studies, to assess the impact of diabetes on its many complications, to avoid the overdiagnosis of diabetes mellitus for insurance and employment reasons, and to aid the practitioner in management of patients.

The terminology, classification, and diagnostic criteria presented in the *Guide* were developed in 1979 by an international work group sponsored by the National Diabetes Data Group of the National Institutes of Health. They have been endorsed by the American Diabetes Association and other major diabetes associations. Changes in the classification and diagnostic criteria are expected as clinical and epidemiologic research reveals more data on various forms of diabetes and other classes of glucose intolerance.

TYPES OF DIABETES MELLITUS AND OTHER CATEGORIES OF GLUCOSE INTOLERANCE

The classification of diabetes mellitus and other categories of glucose intolerance (Table 1) includes three clinical classes and two statistical risk classes that may be part of the natural history of diabetes.

Clinical Classes

The clinical classes of glucose intolerance are *diabetes mellitus, impaired glucose tolerance,* and *gestational diabetes.*

Diabetes Mellitus
Currently, the term *diabetes mellitus* is applied to disorders characterized by fasting hyperglycemia or plasma glucose levels above defined limits during oral glucose tolerance testing. There are three clinical subclasses of diabetes mellitus:

■ **Insulin-dependent (type I) diabetes mellitus**
■ **Non-insulin-dependent (type II) diabetes mellitus**
■ **Other types** (diabetes mellitus associated with certain conditions and syndromes).

Each of these types of diabetes mellitus has distinguishing characteristics.

Type I. Patients with type I diabetes mellitus have severe insulinopenia and are prone to the development of ketoacidosis. Commonly, type I patients are lean and have experienced recent weight loss. By definition, patients with this type of diabetes mellitus are dependent on exogenous insulin to prevent ketoacidosis and death. Type I diabetes is less frequent among some non-White populations and is estimated to account for approximately 10 percent of all known cases of diabetes mellitus. Although type I diabetes may occur at any age, the major peak of onset occurs at about 11 or 12 years, and nearly all patients diagnosed before age 20 are of this type.

Table 1. Types of Diabetes Mellitus and Other Categories of Glucose Intolerance

CLINICAL CLASSES	DISTINGUISHING CHARACTERISTICS
Diabetes mellitus (DM) **Insulin-dependent diabetes mellitus (IDDM) Type I**	Patients may be of any age, are usually thin, and usually have abrupt onset of signs and symptoms with insulinopenia before age 30. These patients often have strongly positive urine ketone tests in conjunction with hyperglycemia and are dependent on insulin therapy to prevent ketoacidosis and to sustain life.
Non-insulin-dependent diabetes mellitus (NIDDM) Type II (obese or nonobese)	Patients usually are older than 30 years at diagnosis, obese, and have relatively few classic symptoms. They are not prone to ketoacidosis except during periods of stress. Although not dependent on exogenous insulin for survival, they may require it for adequate control of hyperglycemia.
Other types of diabetes mellitus	Patients with other types of diabetes mellitus have certain associated conditions or syndromes (see Table 2).
Impaired glucose tolerance (IGT) (obese or nonobese)	Patients with impaired glucose tolerance have plasma glucose levels that are higher than normal but not diagnostic for diabetes mellitus.
Other types of impaired glucose tolerance	Patients with other types of impaired glucose tolerance have certain associated conditions or syndromes (see Table 2).
Gestational diabetes mellitus (GDM)	Patients with gestational diabetes mellitus have onset or discovery of glucose intolerance during pregnancy.
STATISTICAL RISK CLASSES*	
Previous abnormality of glucose tolerance (PreAGT)	Patients in this category have normal glucose tolerance and a history of transient diabetes mellitus or impaired glucose tolerance.
Potential abnormality of glucose tolerance (PotAGT)	Patients in this category have never experienced abnormal glucose tolerance but have a greater than normal risk of developing diabetes mellitus or impaired glucose tolerance.

*Used for epidemiologic and research purposes.

Adapted from classification developed by an international work group sponsored by the National Diabetes Data Group, National Institutes of Health. National Diabetes Data Group: Classification and diagnosis of diabetes mellitus and other categories of glucose intolerance. *Diabetes* 28:1039–57, 1979.

The etiology of type I diabetes mellitus involves immunologic destruction of the beta cells. It appears, however, that it is a heterogeneous disorder in terms of precipitating events. Genetic factors are probably important because there is a clear association between type I diabetes and certain histocompatibility locus antigens (HLA) on chromosome 6. On the other hand, twin studies indicate that only 50 percent of identical twins of type I patients develop the disease. That type I diabetes is an autoimmune disease, is suggested by the observation that the majority of patients have circulating islet cell antibodies at the time of diagnosis. In some patients, acute physiological stress, e.g., viral infections, may precipitate the clinical syndrome.

Type II. Patients with type II diabetes mellitus may have few or none of the classic symptoms of diabetes mellitus when first discovered. Although the symptomatology of type II diabetes mellitus is less obvious than that of type I, this classification of diabetes is also accompanied by vascular and neuropathic complications. In patients with type II diabetes, insulin levels may be normal, depressed, or elevated. Typically, insulin resistance (decreased tissue sensitivity or responsiveness to exogenous and endogenous insulin) is present.

Other characteristics of type II diabetes are as follows.

■ The insulin secretory defects and insulin resistance of type II diabetes are partially reversible.

■ Patients with type II diabetes are not prone to develop ketoacidosis except during periods or conditions of stress, such as those caused by infections, trauma, or surgery.

■ Type II diabetes can occur at any age but is usually diagnosed after age 30.

■ Although about 75 percent of patients are obese or have a history of obesity at the time of diagnosis, type II diabetes can occur in nonobese individuals as well, especially in the elderly.

Although patients with type II diabetes are not dependent on exogenous insulin for survival, many patients require insulin for adequate glycemic control. Insulin may also be needed temporarily for control of stress-induced hyperglycemia (see Pathogenesis).

This type of diabetes accounts for approximately 90 percent of the diabetic patients in the United States. The prevalence of diagnosed type II diabetes mellitus in the United States is about 6 million people, or about 2.5 percent of the population. There probably is an equal number of undiagnosed cases. The prevalence of type II diabetes is markedly increased among American Indians, Blacks, and Hispanics. The prevalence rate increases with age and degree of obesity. There is evidence that the number of new cases diagnosed each year is increasing.

The etiology of type II diabetes mellitus remains unknown. It appears to be a heterogeneous disorder, and genetic and environmental factors seem important. Although type II diabetes mellitus is not associated with specific HLA tissue types, twin studies indicate that there is 90 to 100 percent concordance for this disease in identical twins. There are families in which type II diabetes is present in children, adolescents, and adults and in which an autosomal dominant inheritance has been established. This form of diabetes was formerly referred to as *maturity-onset diabetes of the young* (MODY).

Unlike type I diabetes, circulating islet cell antibodies are rarely present. In-take of excessive calories leading to weight gain and obesity is probably an important factor in the pathogenesis of type II diabetes. In fact, obesity was singled out as the most powerful risk factor by the Expert Committee on Diabetes of the World Health Organization in 1980, and even small weight losses are associated with return of plasma glucose levels toward normal in many patients with this type of diabetes.

Other Types. This category, which is numerically the smallest, includes diabetes mellitus associated with certain diseases or conditions. To be placed in this category, the patient's disease either has to have a known or very likely cause or be part of a specific condition or syndrome. Table 2 presents the several subclasses of this category.

Impaired Glucose Tolerance

Impaired glucose tolerance (IGT) is the term used to describe the condition of individuals who have plasma glucose levels that are higher than normal but lower than those considered diagnostic for diabetes mellitus. Patients in this category may be subgrouped by weight (obese and nonobese). Those with IGT secondary to or associated with certain conditions and syndromes constitute another subgroup (Table 2). It has been shown that about 25 percent of patients with IGT eventually develop diabetes mellitus. Although patients with IGT do not appear to have an increased risk for the microvascular complications of diabetes mellitus, they have been shown in some populations to have a greater than normal risk for atherosclerotic disease.

Gestational Diabetes Mellitus

The term *gestational diabetes mellitus* (GDM) is used to describe glucose intolerance that has its onset or is first detected during pregnancy. Women with known diabetes mellitus before conception are not part of this class. Gestational diabetes occurs in about 2 percent of pregnant women, usually during the second or third trimester, when levels of insulin-antagonist hormones increase and insulin resistance normally occurs. Because fetal morbidity and mortality are increased in the presence of gestational diabetes, it is important to identify women with this condition by performing screening tests in

Table 2. Other Types of Diabetes Mellitus and Impaired Glucose Tolerance

SECONDARY TO:

Pancreatic disease	**Examples:** pancreatectomy, hemochromatosis, cystic fibrosis, chronic pancreatitis
Endocrinopathies	**Examples:** acromegaly, pheochromocytoma, Cushing's syndrome, primary aldosteronism, glucagonoma
Drugs and chemical agents	**Examples:** certain antihypertensive drugs, thiazide diuretics, glucocorticoids, estrogen-containing preparations, psychoactive agents, catecholamines

ASSOCIATED WITH:

Insulin-receptor abnormalities	**Examples:** acanthosis nigricans
Genetic syndromes	**Examples:** hyperlipidemia, muscular dystrophies, Huntington's chorea
Miscellaneous conditions	**Examples:** malnutrition ("tropical diabetes")

For a more complete list, see National Diabetes Data Group: Classification and diagnosis of diabetes mellitus and other categories of glucose tolerance. *Diabetes* 28:1039–57, 1979.

all pregnant women between the 24th and 28th weeks of pregnancy.

After parturition, patients with gestational diabetes should be reclassified on the basis of plasma glucose testing as having diabetes mellitus, impaired glucose tolerance, or a previous abnormality of glucose tolerance (see below). In most cases, glucose tolerance in women with gestational diabetes returns to normal after delivery. Within 5 to 10 years after parturition, however, 30 to 40 percent of women with gestational diabetes develop overt diabetes mellitus (usually type II).

Statistical Risk Classes

There are two classes used to designate stages in the natural history of diabetes mellitus. These statistical risk classes,

which were developed for epidemiologic and research purposes, are *previous abnormality of glucose tolerance* (PrevAGT) and *potential abnormality of glucose tolerance* (PotAGT). Patients now euglycemic, but with previous hyperglycemia in association with prior obesity or during surgical stress, for example, would be classified as PrevAGT. An apparently healthy sibling of an identical twin with type I diabetes mellitus is an example of PotAGT.

DIAGNOSIS OF DIABETES MELLITUS AND OTHER CATEGORIES OF GLUCOSE INTOLERANCE

The prevalence of undiagnosed diabetes mellitus in the United States is about 2.5 percent of the population, and the currently recommended diagnostic tests for diabetes are neither 100 percent specific nor 100 percent sensitive. Based on these facts, it is generally agreed that the risk to the patient of inappropriate diagnosis outweighs the benefits to be gained from indiscriminate screening tests for diabetes.

Indications and Criteria for Screening Tests

Screening tests for diabetes mellitus should be limited to individuals with a high risk that diabetes mellitus is present or likely to develop. Candidates for screening include the following:

■ people with a strong family history of diabetes mellitus,

■ people who are markedly obese,

■ women with a morbid obstetrical history or a history of babies over 9 pounds at birth,

■ all pregnant women between 24 and 28 weeks of pregnancy, and

■ patients with a history of recurrent skin, genital, or urinary tract infections.

It is particularly important to screen all pregnant women for the presence of gestational diabetes, because 60,000 to 90,000 women with gestational diabetes give birth each year, and gestational diabetes is associated with increased perinatal morbidity.

The recommended screening test for nonpregnant adults and children is a fasting plasma glucose level. In pregnant women, a 50-gram oral glucose load is recommended for screening. All women with a history of abnormal glucose tolerance or gestational diabetes should be screened before planned conception. Normal plasma glucose values are presented in Table 3, and criteria for positive screening tests are presented in Table 4.

Indications for Diagnostic Testing

Diagnostic testing should be done only when there are definite indications. Generally accepted indications for diagnostic testing include the following:
■ positive screening test results,
■ the presence of obvious signs and symptoms of diabetes mellitus (polydipsia, polyuria, polyphagia, weight loss), and
■ an incomplete clinical picture such as glycosuria or equivocal elevation of a random plasma glucose level.

Diagnostic Tests for Diabetes Mellitus

When diagnostic testing for diabetes mellitus is indicated, a firm diagnosis should be made on the basis of plasma glucose levels. Although urine glucose tests are strongly suggestive of diabetes in symptomatic patients, they should never be used exclusively for the diagnosis of diabetes mellitus. Furthermore, there are currently insufficient data to support the use of glycosylated protein measurements for the diagnosis of diabetes. The choice of diagnostic tests and their interpretation are different for nonpregnant adults, children, and pregnant women (Table 5).

Tests for diabetes should not be done in the presence of factors that elevate plasma glucose or impair glucose tolerance, such as certain drugs (Tables 2 and 28), stress, marked restriction of carbohydrate intake, or prolonged physical inactivity. Furthermore, drugs and chemicals that may cause lower than normal plasma glucose (e.g., monoamine oxidase inhibitors, propranolol, alcohol, and large quantities of salicylates), as well as those that may elevate plasma glucose levels (e.g., glucocorticosteroids, some oral contraceptives, oral diuretic agents, sympathomimetic agents, beta blockers, and nicotinic acid), should be discontinued, when possible, before testing.

Table 3. Normal Plasma Glucose Values

NONPREGNANT ADULTS	
Fasting plasma glucose	< 115 mg/dl
Plasma glucose values after 75-gram oral glucose dose	30 min < 200 mg/dl 60 min < 200 mg/dl 90 min < 200 mg/dl 120 min < 140 mg/dl
CHILDREN	
Fasting plasma glucose	< 130 mg/dl
Plasma glucose value after glucose dose of 1.75 g/kg ideal body weight up to maximum of 75 grams	120 min < 140 mg/dl

Note: Glucose values above these concentrations but below criteria for diabetes mellitus or impaired glucose tolerance should be considered nondiagnostic.

Criteria for Diagnosis of Diabetes Mellitus

There are differences in the diagnostic criteria for diabetes mellitus in children and in nonpregnant adults. Specifically, criteria for diagnosis in children are more conservative.

Diagnosis in Nonpregnant Adults
In nonpregnant adults, the diagnosis of diabetes mellitus is restricted to those who have *one* of the following:
■ a random plasma glucose level of 200 mg/dl or greater *plus* classic signs and symptoms of diabetes mellitus including polydipsia, polyuria, polyphagia, and weight loss, or
■ a fasting plasma glucose level of 140 mg/dl or greater on at least two occasions. [When the fasting plasma glucose concentration meets this criterion, an oral glucose tolerance test (OGTT) is superfluous because virtually all people with fasting plasma glucose levels of 140 mg/dl or greater will have OGTT results that meet or exceed the diagnostic criteria established for glucose challenge. The OGTT is indicated only if the individual has an indication for

diagnostic testing *and* a fasting plasma glucose level of less than 140 mg/dl.]
- A fasting plasma glucose level of less than 140 mg/dl *plus* sustained elevated plasma glucose levels during at least two OGTTs. Both the 2-hour plasma glucose level and at least one other between 0 and 2 hours after the 75-gram glucose dose must be 200 mg/dl or greater.

Diagnosis in Children

In children, the diagnosis of diabetes mellitus is restricted to those who have *one* of the following:
- a random plasma glucose level of 200 mg/dl or greater *plus* classic signs and symptoms of diabetes mellitus including polyuria, polydipsia, ketonuria, and rapid weight loss, or
- a fasting plasma glucose level of 140 mg/dl or greater on at least two occasions *and* sustained elevated plasma glucose levels during at least two OGTTs. Both the 2-hour plasma glucose and at least one other performed between 0 and 2 hours after the glucose dose (1.75 g/kg ideal body weight up to a maximum of 75 grams) must be 200 mg/dl or greater. The criteria for diagnosis of diabetes

mellitus in an asymptomatic child are very strict. Abnormal glucose tolerance must be documented with at least two elevated fasting plasma glucose levels and at least two abnormal OGTTs. Clearly, there must be a good indication for performing such diagnostic tests in the absence of signs and symptoms of diabetes mellitus.

Oral Glucose Tolerance Test

As noted above, the standard OGTT is usually unnecessary for diagnosis of diabetes mellitus. When indicated, the OGTT is useful only if done with strict adherence to proper methods (see Oral Glucose Tolerance Test, page 9).

Criteria for Diagnosis of Gestational Diabetes

The criteria for diagnosis of gestational diabetes were proposed by O'Sullivan and Mahan in 1964 on the basis of 100-gram OGTTs, and they remain unchanged today. During normal pregnancy, fasting plasma glucose levels tend to fall, and post-glucose-load levels tend to rise. Thus, criteria for diagnosis of gestational diabetes are adjusted appropriately and are calculated to provide maximum sensitivity to diagnose diabetes during pregnancy (Table 5).

EVALUATION AND CLASSIFICATION OF PATIENTS BEFORE TREATMENT

Before therapy is initiated to treat diabetes mellitus or some other type of glucose intolerance, the patient should have a complete medical evaluation and be classified appropriately.

Evaluation of the Patient

A complete evaluation of the patient before therapy helps the physician to classify the patient, to determine the possible presence of underlying diseases that need further study, and to detect the presence of complications frequently associated with diabetes mellitus (see Detection and Treatment of Complications). A reminder list for the evaluation (Office Guide to Initial Evaluation) is presented on page 11.

Classification of the Patient

The patient should not be classified until all data necessary for making the determination are available. Generally, a reasonably good initial assignment of the patient can be made on the basis of diagnostic test results, a complete personal and family history, and complete physical evaluation. The most important distinguishing characteristics of diabetes mellitus and other categories of glucose intolerance are presented in Table 1. Patients should not be classified on the basis of age alone or on the basis of selected therapy.

Special Problems in Classification

There are some special problems in classification that deserve emphasis, the first having to do with IGT.

Impaired Glucose Tolerance vs. Diabetes Mellitus. If diagnostic tests indicate that the patient has IGT, it is important to remember that this type of glucose intolerance does not constitute a definitive diagnosis of diabetes mellitus and that the label of IGT itself may cause problems for the patient with employers and insurance companies. Because the

Oral Glucose Tolerance Test

Although the response to a dose of oral glucose is a sensitive test for diabetes mellitus, it is also fraught with problems in interpretation because it requires strict adherence to detail by the patient and by the person who administers the test.

Patient Selection

Certain patients should be excluded from oral glucose tolerance testing because their responses to glucose challenge will be difficult to interpret, at best, or invalid. For example, this test should not be done on people who are chronically malnourished or on those who have restricted carbohydrate intake to less than 150 grams per day for 3 days or more. People who have been confined to bed for 3 days or more should also be excluded. Test results are invalid in patients experiencing acute medical or surgical stress; such patients probably should not be tested until several months after recovery.

Patient Preparation

The patient should be asked to discontinue medication 3 days before testing when possible and should also be instructed to eat and drink nothing except water for 10 to 14 hours before the test. If the patient normally follows recommendations for a good general diet containing at least 150 grams of carbohydrate a day, a preparatory diet high in carbohydrate is not necessary.

Testing Method

Schedule the test in the morning to exclude diurnal influence on test results. Instruct the patient to refrain from smoking and from drinking coffee just before and during the test. Draw a blood sample for determination of fasting plasma glucose. Give the patient a standard glucose solution (75 grams for nonpregnant adults, 100 grams for pregnant women, and 1.75 g/kg ideal body weight up to 75 grams for children). Ask the patient to remain quiet for the duration of the test (2 hours for children and nonpregnant adults, 3 hours for pregnant women). Start timing when the patient begins to drink the solution, and obtain samples at appropriate intervals. In nonpregnant adults and children, obtain blood samples every 30 minutes for 2 hours. In pregnant women, obtain blood samples every hour for 3 hours.

Table 5. Diagnostic Criteria for Diabetes Mellitus, Impaired Glucose Tolerance, and Gestational Diabetes

NONPREGNANT ADULTS

Criteria for Diabetes Mellitus. Diagnosis of diabetes mellitus in nonpregnant adults should be restricted to those who have *one* of the following:

- random plasma glucose level of 200 mg/dl or greater *plus* classic signs and symptoms of diabetes mellitus including polydipsia, polyuria, polyphagia, and weight loss;

- fasting plasma glucose level of 140 mg/dl or greater on at least 2 occasions; or

- fasting plasma glucose level less than 140 mg/dl *plus* sustained elevated plasma glucose levels during at least 2 oral glucose tolerance tests. The 2-hour sample and at least one other between 0 and 2 hours after 75-gram glucose dose should be 200 mg/dl or greater. Oral glucose tolerance testing is not necessary if patient has fasting plasma glucose level of 140 mg/dl or greater.

Criteria for Impaired Glucose Tolerance. Diagnosis of impaired glucose tolerance in nonpregnant adults should be restricted to those who have *all* of the following:

- fasting plasma glucose of less than 140 mg/dl;

- 2-hour oral glucose tolerance test plasma glucose level between 140 and 200 mg/dl; and

- intervening oral glucose tolerance test plasma glucose level of 200 mg/dl or greater.

PREGNANT WOMEN

Criteria for Gestational Diabetes. After an oral glucose load of 100 grams, diagnosis of gestational diabetes may be made if 2 plasma glucose values equal or exceed (in mg/dl)

Fasting	1 Hour	2 Hour	3 Hour
105	190	165	145

CHILDREN

Criteria for Diabetes Mellitus. Diagnosis of diabetes mellitus in children should be restricted to those who have *one* of the following:

- random plasma glucose level of 200 mg/dl or greater *plus* classic signs and symptoms of diabetes mellitus, including polyuria, polydipsia, ketonuria, and rapid weight loss; or

- fasting plasma glucose level of 140 mg/dl or greater on at least 2 occasions *and* sustained elevated plasma glucose levels during at least 2 oral glucose tolerance tests. Both the 2-hour plasma glucose and at least one other between 0 and 2 hours after glucose dose (1.75 g/kg ideal body weight up to 75 grams) should be 200 mg/dl or greater.

Criteria for Impaired Glucose Tolerance. Diagnosis of impaired glucose tolerance in children should be restricted to those who have *both* of the following:

- fasting plasma glucose concentration of less than 140 mg/dl; and

- 2-hour oral glucose tolerance test plasma glucose level of greater than 140 mg/dl.

finding of IGT may identify a person with higher than normal risk of developing diabetes and atherosclerotic heart disease, most physicians continue to regularly observe the patient. If the patient with IGT is obese, attention should be given to weight control and to modification of vascular risk factors.

Type I vs. Type II Diabetes Mellitus. Another major problem in classification is that it is sometimes difficult to assign the patient to a particular subclass of diabetes mellitus (i.e., type I vs. type II). For example, the thin type II patient who has been taking insulin often looks like a type I patient. Another example is the newly diagnosed child or adolescent who is a member of a family with an autosomal dominant form of inheritance of diabetes. This patient usually has type II diabetes and should not be classified as type I on the basis of age alone. Finally, there are patients with characteristics of type II diabetes who may require insulin therapy for glycemic control but are not dependent on it to prevent ketoacidosis or to sustain life. These patients should not be classified as type I simply on the basis of insulin therapy.

Currently, it is not necessary for clinicians to measure islet cell antibodies or the degree of insulin secretion. In research studies, measurement of plasma C-peptide after an oral stimulus is often used as an index of insulin secretion; however, it has not proved to be a useful classification tool. In the future, reliable measurements of islet cell antibodies may be useful in the classification of diabetes. Currently, a history of ketoacidosis or the detection of moderate to strong urine ketones in the presence of hyperglycemia is the most useful indicator of type I diabetes mellitus. Although the classification of some patients may thus be problematic, the goal of therapy remains the achievement of euglycemia.

Reclassification of the Patient

After therapy is initiated, the patient should be reevaluated from time to time and reclassified accordingly. In this regard, it is important to reemphasize that the specific therapy used to treat a patient is not the determining factor in classification.

BIBLIOGRAPHY

Bennett PH: The diagnosis of diabetes: new international classification and diagnostic criteria. *Annu Rev Med* 34:295–309, 1983

Freinkel N (Ed.): Proceedings of the Second International Workshop-Conference on Gestational Diabetes Mellitus. *Diabetes* 34: Suppl. 2, 1985

Genuth S: Classification and diagnosis of diabetes mellitus. *Clinical Diabetes* 1:1–20, 1983

Keen H: Limitations and problems of diabetes classification from an epidemiological point of view. *Adv Exp Med Biol* 189:31–46, 1985

National Diabetes Data Group: Classification and diagnosis of diabetes mellitus and other categories of glucose intolerance. *Diabetes* 28: 1039–57, 1979

O'Sullivan JB, Mahan CM: Criteria for the oral glucose tolerance test in pregnancy. *Diabetes* 13:278–85, 1964

Simon D, Coignet H, Thibult N: Comparison of glycosylated hemoglobin and fasting plasma glucose with two-hour post-load plasma glucose in the detection of diabetes mellitus. *Am J Epidemiol* 122:589–93, 1985

Office Guide to Initial Evaluation

Before therapy for diabetes mellitus is begun, the patient should have a complete evaluation, including a search for the presence of complications frequently associated with diabetes (see Detection and Treatment of Complications). The following is a reminder list for the complete initial evaluation.

General Evaluation

Routine history
Routine physical examination
Determination of ideal body weight
(see Management)

Glycemic Control

Fasting plasma glucose
Glycosylated hemoglobin

Evaluation for Complications

Visual impairment
    Ophthalmic examination
Nephropathy
    Complete urinalysis (including protein)
    Blood urea nitrogen
    Serum creatinine
Neuropathy
    Neurologic examination
Accelerated atherosclerotic disease
    Serum cholesterol, high-density lipoprotein cholesterol
    Serum triglycerides
    Electrocardiogram
    Peripheral pulses, bruits
Leg/foot ulcers and cutaneous problems
    Foot and skin examination

Pathogenesis of Type II Diabetes Mellitus

Highlights

Non-insulin-dependent (type II) diabetes mellitus is a heterogeneous disorder characterized by impaired beta-cell function and diminished tissue (liver, muscle, and adipose tissue) sensitivity to insulin.

In type II diabetes
- basal insulin secretion is normal or increased;
- glucose-stimulated insulin secretion is often normal or increased when viewed in absolute terms; however, relative to the degree of hyperglycemia, insulin secretion is impaired;
- insulin resistance is usually present;
- tissue sensitivity to insulin and beta-cell secretion are in a dynamic state of flux; and

- an initial defect in tissue sensitivity to insulin can lead to the emergence of a defect in insulin secretion; conversely, an impairment in beta-cell function can lead to a disturbance in insulin action (Figure 1, page 18).

By the time most patients with type II diabetes come to medical attention, significant fasting hyperglycemia is present, and defects in insulin action and insulin secretion are well established.

Once the full-blown diabetic syndrome is established, it is impossible to determine in any given individual whether the primary defect originated in the beta cell or in peripheral tissues.

Pathogenesis of Type II Diabetes Mellitus

INTRODUCTION

Non-insulin-dependent (type II) diabetes mellitus is a heterogeneous disorder characterized by impaired beta-cell function and diminished tissue (liver and muscle) sensitivity to insulin. There has been considerable debate as to which defect (i.e., impaired insulin secretion or impaired insulin action) is the initial lesion in the pathogenesis of type II diabetes. It is clear, however, that both insulin secretion and insulin action are markedly impaired in diabetic individuals who have had the disease for any significant length of time and who have moderately severe fasting hyperglycemia (plasma glucose >180–200 mg/dl).

In recent years, a significant body of evidence has accumulated that indicates that defects in insulin secretion can lead to insulin resistance and vice versa. Thus, once the full-blown diabetic syndrome has become established, it is impossible to determine in any given individual whether the primary defect originated in the beta cell or in peripheral/hepatic tissues.

Obviously, more information about the relationship between abnormalities in insulin secretion and insulin action is needed for a full understanding of type II diabetes mellitus. Nonetheless, certain general statements about the pathogenesis of type II diabetes can be made.

INSULIN SECRETION

In nondiabetic individuals, there are two phases of insulin release: (1) an early phase that occurs within the first 30 minutes after glucose ingestion and that represents the release of insulin stored within the beta cell and (2) a later phase of insulin secretion that includes newly synthesized insulin.

Fasting Insulin Concentration

Patients with type II diabetes mellitus usually have normal or elevated fasting plasma insulin levels. This postabsorptive hyperinsulinemia reflects an augmented basal rate of insulin secretion that occurs in response to elevated fasting plasma glucose concentrations. The latter, however, is less than nondiabetic individuals would have if their plasma glucose levels were comparably increased.

The fasting insulin level is diminished only when marked fasting hyperglycemia (>250–300 mg/dl) occurs. When this happens, beta-cell function is severely disturbed, and the patient more closely resembles an individual with insulin-dependent (type I) diabetes mellitus. As will be discussed, this fasting hyperinsulinemia may play an important role in the subsequent development of insulin resistance.

Glucose-Stimulated Insulin Response

In individuals with impaired glucose tolerance* and fasting plasma glucose levels of less than 115 mg/dl, the total plasma insulin response after oral or intravenous glucose administration is normal or, more often, elevated. When the fasting plasma glucose concentration exceeds 115 mg/dl in an individual with impaired glucose tolerance, the early phase of insulin secretion becomes markedly diminished, and the late phase of insulin secretion remains normal or, more often, is increased.

In diabetic patients with moderate fasting hyperglycemia (140–180 mg/dl), the late phase of insulin secretion usually remains within the normal range. Because these individuals are markedly insulin resistant (see subsequent discussion), a "normal" plasma insulin response is, in fact, quite abnormal and inadequate to maintain normal glucose tolerance. In nondiabetic individuals,

---

The diagnostic criteria for impaired glucose tolerance and for diabetes mellitus are presented in Table 5 (see page 10).

the presence of insulin resistance (such as in obesity) is compensated for by an increase in insulin secretion. As the diabetic state progressively worsens and more severe hyperglycemia (>180–200 mg/dl) ensues, the plasma insulin response to both intravenous and oral glucose becomes negligible. Diabetic individuals with fasting plasma glucose levels between 120 and 180 mg/dl may have increased, normal, or decreased plasma insulin responses to hyperglycemia. Within this range, however, patients with the highest fasting plasma glucose concentrations tend to have diminished insulin secretion, whereas those with the lowest glucose levels usually demonstrate normal to increased beta-cell insulin secretion.

Physiologic Consequences of Impaired Insulin Secretion

The impairment in insulin secretion has important physiologic consequences. When the early phase of insulin release is inhibited, the portal vein insulin concentration remains low and hepatic glucose production is not suppressed. Continued endogenous output of glucose by the liver, supplemented by glucose entering the circulation via the gastrointestinal tract, leads to excessive hyperglycemia, which, in turn, leads to enhanced secretion of insulin during the hours after glucose ingestion. Eventually, the plasma glucose concentration will return to normal but only at the expense of the resultant late hyperinsulinemia.

As the defect in beta-cell secretion becomes more severe, the late phase of insulin secretion is diminished. When this happens, fasting hyperglycemia and abnormal glucose tolerance develop, and the severity of the glucose intolerance closely parallels the defect in insulin secretion.

Summary

In type II diabetes mellitus, beta-cell function is impaired, but in response to fasting hyperglycemia, basal insulin secretion is normal or increased. In individuals with impaired glucose tolerance, the total plasma insulin response to a glucose challenge is usually increased, even though the early insulin response

is lost when the fasting plasma glucose concentration exceeds 115 to 120 mg/dl. If moderate to severe fasting hyperglycemia (>180–200 mg/dl) is present, all phases of insulin secretion are markedly impaired. With intermediate fasting plasma glucose levels (120–180 mg/dl), the plasma insulin response to glucose may be increased, normal, or decreased and, in general, is inversely correlated with the degree of fasting hyperglycemia.

INSULIN RESISTANCE

It is well established that insulin resistance is an early defect and present in the vast majority of individuals with impaired glucose tolerance and essentially in all patients with type II diabetes mellitus who have fasting plasma glucose levels of 140 mg/dl or greater. An impairment in endogenous insulin action was first suggested by the observation that many patients with type II diabetes have normal or increased plasma insulin responses after glucose ingestion but are glucose intolerant. Subsequently, numerous investigators, with a variety of different experimental techniques, have demonstrated the nearly uniform presence of insulin resistance in type II diabetes. The insulin resistance is positively correlated with the elevation in fasting plasma glucose concentration. Thus, individuals with greater glucose intolerance are more insulin resistant than those with lesser degrees of glucose intolerance.

Sites of Insulin Resistance

Numerous studies demonstrate that insulin resistance exists in both hepatic and peripheral tissues. Whereas this discussion focuses on the consequences of insulin resistance on glucose metabolism, it should be acknowledged that insulin has important effects on a variety of other metabolic processes, abnormalities of which may have important consequences, particularly in the development of the complications of diabetes. Impairment in muscle glucose uptake results from diminished glucose oxidation as well as impaired nonoxidative pathways of glucose utilization, primarily glycogen formation. This decrease in insulin-mediated muscle glucose disposal contributes to the excessive rise in plasma glucose concentration after glucose injection.

Despite the presence of fasting hyperinsulinemia, basal rates of hepatic glucose production are uniformly increased when the fasting plasma glucose concentration exceeds 140 mg/dl. Furthermore, the increase in basal hepatic glucose production is strongly correlated with the level of fasting plasma glucose. When insulin is infused, patients with type II diabetes fail to demonstrate a normal suppression of hepatic glucose output.

Mechanisms of Insulin Resistance at Cellular Level

In the most general sense, the action of insulin involves two processes. First, insulin binds to a specific receptor located on the cell surface. Second, this interaction activates a series of intracellular events, including enhanced glucose transport and stimulation of a variety of intracellular enzymatic pathways. For the sake of simplicity, all the intracellular processes involved in insulin action after it binds to its receptor will be referred to as postbinding events.

Binding Abnormalities

Insulin binding to monocytes and erythrocytes in individuals with impaired glucose tolerance and in individuals with mild fasting hyperglycemia may be reduced. This reduction in binding results from a decrease in insulin receptor number without any change in receptor affinity. However, because most patients with type II diabetes mellitus are obese and hyperinsulinemic, this decreased binding may be secondary to obesity and hyperinsulinemia. Recent studies on liver and adipose tissue have demonstrated normal or only slightly reduced insulin binding. Thus, a decrease in insulin binding is unlikely to play a major role in the insulin resistance of type II diabetes. However, the insulin receptor has functions (e.g., enzymatic) in addition to hormone binding; abnormalities of which may contribute to this resistance.

Postbinding Abnormalities

Postbinding abnormalities are primarily responsible for the insulin resistance in patients with type II diabetes who have significant fasting hyperglycemia (>140 mg/dl). As noted above, some investigators who have examined insulin binding to adipocytes obtained from type II diabetic patients have been unable to demonstrate any decrease in either receptor number or affinity. Nonetheless, they have demonstrated a marked decrease in glucose transport and other intracellular processes involved in glucose metabolism. Furthermore, in vivo studies have shown that transport of glucose into the cell as well as a number of other intracellular processes involved in glucose metabolism are impaired.

Summary

In patients with type II diabetes, postbinding abnormalities are primarily responsible for the insulin resistance; impaired insulin binding when present may be secondary to associated obesity and hyperinsulinemia but, nevertheless, may also contribute to impaired tissue insulin sensitivity.

PATHOGENETIC SEQUENCES LEADING TO TYPE II DIABETES MELLITUS

By the time most patients with type II diabetes mellitus come to medical attention, significant fasting hyperglycemia is present, and defects in insulin action and insulin secretion are well established. With current knowledge, it is difficult to know which defect occurred first in the natural history of the disease. What seems to be evolving as a common theme is that abnormalities in insulin secretion can lead to the development of insulin resistance, and, conversely, an impairment in glucose uptake by peripheral tissues may secondarily eventuate in beta-cell failure. The interrelationship between the two principal mechanisms (i.e., impaired insulin secretion and insulin resistance) responsible for glucose intolerance in type II diabetes is presented in Figure 1 (page 18).

Primary Beta-Cell Defect

In essentially all patients with type II diabetes, the insulin secretory response

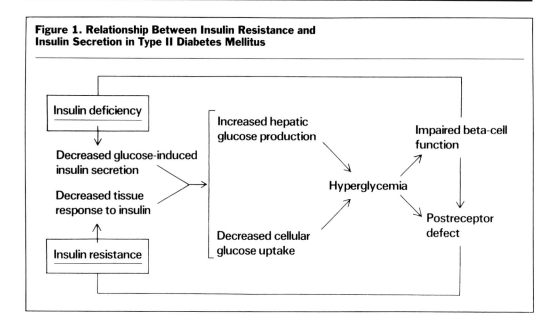

Figure 1. Relationship Between Insulin Resistance and Insulin Secretion in Type II Diabetes Mellitus

to glucose is delayed, and in many it is absolutely diminished (Figure 1). This defective insulin secretory response leads to inadequate suppression of hepatic glucose production and a decrease in glucose uptake by peripheral tissues during the period immediately after glucose ingestion. The resulting postprandial hyperglycemia provides a persistent stimulus to insulin secretion, and the resultant hyperinsulinemia will eventually return the plasma glucose concentration to normal. However, fasting euglycemia will be maintained only at the expense of an increased plasma insulin concentration.

It is well established that insulin is the most important factor involved in the regulation of its own receptor. Thus, chronic hyperinsulinemia will cause a downregulation of the number of insulin receptors. Chronic hyperinsulinemia can also lead to postbinding defects. Both of these mechanisms can lead to the development of insulin resistance.

The clinical counterpart of this pathogenetic sequence is a patient with impaired glucose tolerance. This individual is characterized by a decreased early plasma insulin response to glucose, a normal or increased total plasma insulin response, reduced insulin binding, impaired suppression of hepatic glucose production, and reduced peripheral glucose uptake. Postbinding alterations in glucose utilization may be present.

As the insulin response to glucose be-

comes progressively more deficient, fasting hyperglycemia occurs. The progressive nature of the insulin secretory abnormality may result from several factors: (1) the natural history of the beta-cell defect, which is genetically determined; (2) persistent hyperglycemia, which has detrimental effects on the beta cell and causes a progressive impairment in insulin secretion; or (3) some other, as yet unrecognized, metabolic disturbance that is present in the diabetic milieu.

As beta-cell function becomes progressively impaired, the insulin secretory response becomes deficient, and a major postbinding defect in insulin action emerges. In the basal state, the majority (~70 percent) of glucose is taken up by insulin-independent tissues, primarily brain, and therefore, the major factor responsible for fasting hyperglycemia is increased hepatic glucose production. After glucose ingestion, however, insulin-dependent tissues (primarily muscle and liver) are largely responsible for the disposal of the glucose load. Thus, when the beta-cell response becomes absolutely diminished, marked postbinding abnormalities (i.e., glucose transport and intracellular glucose metabolism) develop. The development of fasting hyperglycemia further aggravates the insulin resistance.

The clinical picture that emerges from the sequence of events just described is typical of the patient with type II diabetes. Both the early and late phases of insulin secretion are impaired, and marked peripheral tissue (muscle) insulin resistance is present. Although some patients may have diminished insulin binding, postbinding abnormalities are primarily responsible for the defect in insulin action. Such individuals with type II diabetes have elevated rates of basal hepatic glucose production, reduced basal rates of glucose clearance, and impaired ability of insulin to suppress hepatic glucose output and increase glucose utilization.

The preceding sequence of events has been directly validated by experimental observations: when dogs or rats are rendered partially diabetic by alloxan, streptozocin, or partial pancreatectomy, moderate to severe muscle and hepatic resistance to the action of insulin develops.

Primary Cellular Defect

From the preceding discussion, it can be reasoned that a primary defect at the cellular level would also lead to the development of an abnormality in insulin secretion and the typical picture of type II diabetes (Figure 1). In some normal-weight diabetic individuals with mild fasting hyperglycemia, and in most obese type II diabetic patients (who account for approximately 75 percent of the adult diabetic population), insulin secretion is increased compared with nonobese control subjects with normal glucose tolerance. The disturbance in glucose metabolism in these patients is best described as a primary cellular defect (binding or postbinding) in insulin-mediated glucose metabolism. The insulin resistance by itself is sufficient to reduce glucose uptake, increase hepatic glucose production, or both. This results in a small increment in the fasting plasma glucose concentration. The normal response of a beta cell is for it to augment its secretion of insulin in an attempt to return the plasma glucose concentration to normal.

Overfeeding studies have clearly established that weight gain uniformly leads to the development of insulin resistance in lean subjects with previously normal insulin sensitivity. However, the insulin resistance, in and of itself, initially does not lead to fasting hyperglycemia, because the healthy beta cell is able to appropriately augment its secretion of insulin to maintain normal glucose.

As insulin resistance becomes more severe in the obese individual susceptible to diabetes, fasting hyperglycemia develops despite an augmented (but insufficient) rate of insulin secretion. The resultant hyperinsulinemia further exacerbates the insulin resistance. With time, the beta cells can no longer maintain their augmented rate of insulin secretion, progressive insulin deficiency ensues, and postbinding defects in insulin action emerge (or become worse). The precise mechanism(s) responsible for development of impaired insulin secretion are currently unknown.

The sequence of events outlined above is particularly characteristic of the obese patient with type II diabetes. Obesity per se is known to be associated with marked insulin resistance. Nonetheless, glucose tolerance usually remains normal because of an augmented insulin response. Only after the beta cell begins to exhaust does overt fasting hyperglycemia develop in obese individuals.

Summary

In summary, both tissue sensitivity to insulin and beta-cell secretion are in a dynamic state of flux in type II diabetes mellitus. Insulin resistance can lead to the development of a defect in insulin secretion, and, similarly, impaired beta-cell function can lead to a disturbance in insulin action. This explains why both insulin resistance and impaired insulin secretion are so uniformly observed in type II diabetes once the full-blown diabetic syndrome is established.

BIBLIOGRAPHY

Campbell PJ, Mandarino LJ, Gerich J: Quantification of the relative impairments in actions of insulin on hepatic glucose production and peripheral glucose uptake in NIDDM. *Metabolism* 32:151–56, 1988

DeFronzo RA: The triumvirate—β-cell, liver, and muscle: a collusion responsible for type II diabetes mellitus. *Diabetes.* In press

DeFronzo RA, Ferrannini E, Koivisto V: New concepts in the pathogenesis and treatment of noninsulin-dependent diabetes mellitus. *Am J Med* 74 (Suppl. 1A):52–81, 1983

Reaven GM: Insulin resistance in noninsulin-dependent diabetes mellitus: does it exist and can it be measured? *Am J Med* 74 (Suppl. 1A):3–17, 1983

Management of Type II Diabetes Mellitus

Highlights

THERAPEUTIC OBJECTIVES AND PLAN

The two major goals of management of type II diabetes mellitus are to
- achieve normal metabolic biochemical control and
- prevent vascular complications

Recommendations for the Biochemical Indices of Metabolic Control are shown on page 25.

The three recommended treatment modalities are
- dietary modification,
- increased physical activity, and
- pharmacologic intervention with either an oral hypoglycemic agent or insulin.

Patient education is necessary for the successful management of type II diabetes mellitus.

DIETARY MODIFICATION

Modification of the diet is the most important element in the therapeutic plan for patients with type II diabetes, and, for some patients, it is the only intervention needed to control the metabolic abnormalities associated with the disease.

When the patient is overweight, total caloric intake should be decreased.

Significant caloric restriction usually is successful in lowering plasma glucose levels even before significant weight loss is achieved.

Daily caloric requirements and various approaches to weight reduction are outlined on page 27.

Calories should be spread as evenly as possible throughout the major daily meals. In general, meals taken 4 to 5 hours apart allow adequate time for the postprandial glucose concentration to return to preprandial levels.

Recommendations for nutrient content of the diet, including protein, simple and complex carbohydrates, fat, and dietary fiber are presented on pages 28 and 29.

Patients with diabetes have greater than normal prevalence of hyperlipidemia, atherosclerosis, and hypertension. Dietary recommendations related to these conditions should be observed (page 29).

The use of alcohol and nonnutritive sweeteners is discussed on page 30.

Implementation of a specific meal plan requires
- patient education and often behavior modification and
- individualization of the meal plan.

The help of a qualified nutritionist or dietitian facilitates successful dietary management.

The major deterrents to successful diet therapy are summarized in Table 8, page 32.

APPROPRIATE PHYSICAL ACTIVITY

Unless contraindicated, appropriate physical activity should be recommended as an adjunct to dietary modification.

The potential benefits of increased physical activity include
- improvement in insulin sensitivity and possible improvement in glucose tolerance,
- promotion of weight loss and maintenance of ideal body weight when combined with restricted caloric intake,
- amelioration of cardiovascular risk factors,
- potential reduction in dosage or need for insulin or oral hypoglycemic agents,
- enhancement of work capacity, and
- enrichment of quality of life and improvement in sense of well-being.

For some patients, there are potential hazards associated with increased physical activity, including hypoglycemia during or after exercise (page 33).

Exercise should not be prescribed if the patient has poorly controlled, labile blood glucose levels or is at increased risk because of diabetic complications.

Complete guidelines for the exercise prescription are presented on pages 34 and 35.

PHARMACOLOGIC INTERVENTION

When the patient cannot achieve normal or near-normal plasma glucose levels with dietary modification and regular exercise, pharmacologic intervention should be considered.

Pharmacologic intervention is an adjunct to and not a substitute for dietary modification and exercise.

The choice between oral hypoglycemic agent and insulin should be made with the particular patient in mind, taking into account
- the total clinical context of the patient's disease,
- the patient's acceptance of the various therapeutic modalities,
- the patient's level of diabetes education, and
- the patient's motivation.

A general guide is presented in Table 14, page 45.

Oral agents augment beta-cell insulin secretion acutely. After several months, insulin levels return to pretreatment values while glucose levels remain improved, which suggests that sulfonylurea agents exert extra pancreatic as well as pancreatic effects on glucose metabolism.

The currently available FDA-approved sulfonylurea agents differ from one another in terms of potency, pharmacokinetics, and metabolism (Table 10, page 38).

Approximately 60 to 70 percent of patients with type II diabetes will demonstrate an initial satisfactory response to sulfonylurea therapy.

The patient who is most likely to respond to oral agents
- has had onset of diabetes after 40 years of age,
- has had diabetes for fewer than 5 years and is normal weight or obese,
- has never received insulin or has been well controlled on less than 40 units per day.

About 5 to 20 percent of patients experience secondary failure, which may be due to failure of the patient to follow the prescribed dietary plan, progression of disease, or the occurrence of an underlying stressful disease or condition.

Oral agents are contraindicated if the patient
- has type I diabetes,
- is pregnant or lactating,
- has a stressful concurrent condition with significant hyperglycemia,
- is allergic to sulfonylurea compounds.

Side effects of oral agents are relatively uncommon. The major complication of sulfonylurea therapy is hypoglycemia. Elderly patients are more susceptible to hypoglycemia induced by oral agents, particularly when they have a tendency to skip meals and when liver, renal, or cardiovascular function is impaired. Very potent and longer-acting sulfonylureas should be used with caution in these individuals.

Factors that influence the choice of agent are outlined on page 37. When prescribing an oral agent, the lowest effective dose should be used initially, and the dose should be increased every 1 or 2 weeks until desired glycemic control is achieved or until the maximum dose is reached.

It is possible for insulin to achieve satisfactory blood glucose control in patients with type II diabetes. However, the insulin resistance of some patients—particularly those who are obese—may be very difficult to overcome and may require large quantities of insulin.

Several circumstances demand the use of insulin in type II diabetic patients, such as

- periods of acute injury, infection, or surgery,
- pregnancy,
- allergy or serious reaction to sulfonylurea agents.

Human and pork insulins are usually more expensive than beef or mixed beef/pork standard insulins and are indicated for patients with insulin allergy, severe insulin resistance due to insulin antibodies, lipoatrophy, onset of diabetes during pregnancy, or acute problems that require intermittent insulin therapy.

The insulin prescription depends on the desired course of action (Table 13, page 43). Some patients with mild to moderate fasting hyperglycemia may be adequately controlled with one injection of intermediate-acting insulin before breakfast. Many patients require a regimen consisting of short-acting insulin in combination with either intermediate-acting or long-acting insulin (Figure 2, page 44).

The complications of insulin therapy include hypoglycemia, lipodystrophies, antibody formation including insulin resistance, and allergy (both local and systemic). These complications may be managed by changing the dose or type of insulin.

Currently, the only candidate for treatment with both insulin and an oral hypoglycemic agent is the unusual patient in whom glycemic control cannot be achieved with diet and sulfonylurea therapy and in whom reasonable glycemic control cannot be achieved with insulin alone. The efficacy of combination therapy for such patients has not been established, and referral to a specialist is recommended.

SPECIAL THERAPEUTIC PROBLEMS: PREGNANCY AND SURGERY

Ideally, pregnancy in a patient with diabetes should be planned so that conception occurs when the patient has normal fasting, preprandial, and postprandial plasma glucose levels. Consultation with personnel at a regionalized tertiary care program should be sought before conception. Goals for glycemic control are outlined on page 46. Referral should be considered if the plasma glucose level exceeds 120 mg/dl at any time during pregnancy.

The major principles governing the management of diabetic patients during surgery are presented in Table 15, page 47. The objectives of management before, during, and after surgery are to prevent hypoglycemia and hyperglycemia.

ASSESSMENT OF TREATMENT

The therapeutic response to treatment of diabetes mellitus is monitored by determining effects on glucose metabolism.
Physicians monitor the responses to treatment with determinations of fasting, preprandial, and postprandial plasma glucose levels (an index of day-to-day control) and with assays for glycosylated hemoglobin (a reflection of degree of glucose control for the preceding 2 months).

Patients can determine the effects of therapy by self-monitoring of blood glucose and measurement of urine ketones when necessary. They can use a daily journal to record food intake, meal plan, doses of insulin or oral hypoglycemic agent, symptoms, and results of self-administered urine and blood tests.

Self-monitoring of blood glucose makes it possible for some patients to achieve euglycemia, and it provides assurance against hypoglycemia.

Products for self-monitoring of blood glucose are presented in Table 16, page 49.

Management of Type II Diabetes Mellitus

THERAPEUTIC OBJECTIVES AND PLAN

A rational approach to the treatment of patients with non-insulin-dependent (type II) diabetes mellitus should include measures that will specifically reverse the underlying pathogenetic metabolic disturbances that result in fasting hyperglycemia—namely, insulin resistance and impaired beta-cell function. When a treatment plan designed to achieve normalization of plasma glucose concentration is successfully employed, it is hoped that the result of long-term glycemic control will be prevention or amelioration of the major complications of diabetes mellitus, e.g., accelerated atherosclerosis (the macroangiopathy of diabetes), diabetes-specific microvascular complications (the microangiopathy of diabetes leading to retinopathy and nephropathy), neuropathic disease, and infection (see Detection and Treatment of Complications).

The prevention of microvascular complications by tight glucose control has been clearly established in animal models. Preliminary data in humans support this concept but are not conclusive. Although long-term benefits of glucose control have not been unequivocally demonstrated, it is logical and prudent to attempt to reduce blood glucose levels to normal if such attempts are not grossly disturbing to the life-style of the patient.

There are two major goals of management for the type II diabetic patient: (1) to achieve normal metabolic biochemical control and (2) to prevent vascular complications. To achieve the first goal, the physician adjusts management to produce normal levels of fasting and postprandial plasma glucose, of fasting cholesterol and triglycerides, and of glycosylated hemoglobin. To prevent vascular complications, it is important not only to achieve the first goal, but also to lower elevated blood pressure to normal and help the patient to stop smoking and achieve desirable body weight.

A variety of approaches may be used to achieve these goals of management. First, it is critical to educate the patient and his/her family about diabetes mellitus. National standards now exist for diabetes education programs, and these should be followed. In addition, a diabetic meal plan and exercise program should be developed. Therapeutic decisions about diet and pharmacologic therapy should be made, and a program should be instituted to make an accurate assessment of metabolic control. Within this scheme, careful attention to psychosocial influences and/or behavior

Biochemical Indices of Metabolic Control: Top Limits

BIOCHEMICAL INDEX	NORMAL	ACCEPTABLE	POOR
Fasting plasma glucose	115	140	>200 mg/dl
Postprandial (2-hr) plasma glucose	140	200	>235 mg/dl
Glycosylated hemoglobin	6	8	>10%
Fasting plasma cholesterol	200	<240	>240 mg/dl
Fasting plasma triglyceride	150	200	>250 mg/dl

Adjust for normal values of laboratory.

modification techniques are exceptionally valuable. Finally, the physican must have indices that indicate results of attempts at metabolic control (see Biochemical Indices of Metabolic Control, page 25). Although it is recognized that normal levels may not always be achieved, this remains the goal of optimal therapy. Of course, plasma glucose goals should not be achieved at the expense of recurrent episodes of severe hypoglycemia. Note that laboratory values may differ from those in the indices, particularly for glycosylated hemoglobin and lipids, depending on the methods used.

If the physician accepts these goals of management, follows the suggested approaches, uses indices of biochemical management, and strives to correct the vascular risk factors of obesity, hypertension, and cigarette smoking, he/she will contribute significantly to an improved life-style and the prevention or delay of vascular complications in type II diabetic patients.

Dietary Modification

Modification of the diet is the most important element in the therapeutic plan for patients with type II diabetes mellitus. In fact, for some patients, prescription of an appropriate diet is the only therapeutic intervention needed to effectively control the metabolic abnormalities associated with this disease.

Dietary therapy is concerned with the following:
■ maintenance of proper nutrition,
■ total number of calories ingested,
■ individual food sources that make up these calories, and
■ distribution of calories throughout the day.

Unfortunately, there is no formula for dietary modification that applies to all patients with type II diabetes mellitus. Thus, no handout diet sheet can be used as a substitute for planning and supervising dietary modification. In fact, it is the unusual physician who can design and prescribe a dietary plan that achieves the desired results without help from a trained dietitian or nutritionist.

In most communities, physicians can find a health-care professional in a hospital or in private practice who is willing and qualified to help with this aspect of therapy. In many cases, a local American Diabetes Association affiliate (see listing on pages 95–98) can provide the necessary information or back-up nutritional support.

Importance of Patient Cooperation/ Professional Support

It is obvious that patient cooperation is the key to successful execution of prescribed dietary modification. What may not be so obvious is that the patient must be consulted in the planning stage to ensure that the dietary plan is one that can be embraced with enthusiasm. It has been shown that patients are more likely to adhere to dietary prescriptions if they understand the importance of, and help to devise, dietary modifications.

Helping the patient to achieve the goals of dietary therapy requires instruction, encouragement, frequent follow-up evaluation and education, and, in many instances, behavior modification therapy (see Techniques for Helping the Patient Cope With Diagnosis and Treatment, page 57). Unless the physician has an abundance of free time, it is best to merely define the dietary objectives and to leave the specifics of the plan and its execution to a trained nutritionist or dietitian.

Therapeutic Goals and General Principles

When a dietary plan is prescribed for the patient, the important considerations include the patient's nutritional requirements and daily caloric needs as well as the distribution of calories throughout the day and the nutrient content of the diet.

Nutritional Requirements. The nutritional requirements of the patient with type II diabetes are basically the same as those of the general population. An excellent resource for general nutritional guidelines and information is the American Diabetes Association's *Nutritional Recommendations and Principles for Individuals with Diabetes Mellitus, 1986.*

Total Caloric Intake. Because most patients with type II diabetes are overweight, caloric restriction is important and can be of great benefit. Significant caloric restriction is usually successful in lowering plasma glucose levels even before significant weight loss is achieved. Depending on the degree of obesity present initially and the amount of weight loss, sustained beneficial effects on glycemic control can be maintained after the goal weight is achieved and a eucaloric diet is initiated. In general, the more recent the onset of type II diabetes, the more responsive the patient will be to the beneficial effects of weight reduction.

Weight loss leads to a reduction in the accelerated rates of hepatic glucose production and ameliorates the degree of insulin resistance by increasing insulin receptors and reducing the magnitude of the postreceptor defect in insulin action. Weight loss may also improve beta-cell secretion.

Motivated patients can usually lose weight successfully during the initial dietary period, but it is the unusual patient who keeps the pounds off. The major challenge in weight reduction therapy is to develop a proper supportive environment and patient motivation to maintain weight loss after it has been achieved. Consideration should be given to encouraging overweight patients with diabetes to utilize support groups such as Weight Watchers, TOPS, and Overeaters Anonymous.

Daily Caloric Requirement. There are many ways to calculate daily caloric expenditure, but the average normal man expends about 35 kcal/kg body weight per day; 25 kcal/kg body weight is attributed to the basal metabolic rate, the rest to physical activity and the thermal effect of food. Sedentary individuals need about 30 kcal/kg body weight per day; moderately active individuals need around 35 kcal/kg body weight per day. For those who engage in brisk physical exertion for prolonged intervals throughout the day, caloric expenditure can exceed 35 kcal/kg body weight.

Another factor that affects caloric requirements (at least on a per kilogram basis) is the degree of adiposity. Adipose tissue is predominantly storage triglyceride, which is relatively inert metabolically, with a decreased caloric need per unit weight. Thus, the greater the degree of adiposity, the lower the caloric requirements per kilogram.

The essential tenet of weight reduction is straightforward. If caloric expenditure exceeds intake, weight will be lost. On average, a total caloric deficit of 3,500 kilocalories will lead to a tissue weight loss of 1 pound.

Various Approaches to Weight Reduction. There are a number of approaches to weight reduction. Basically, they differ from one another in degree of caloric restriction and rate of weight loss, dietary constituents, and the employment of behavioral and psychological support measures. Among the approaches we recommend are the following:
■ nutritionally sound, modestly restricted diets that achieve slow, gradual weight loss over several months;
■ increased physical activity;
■ behavior modification; and
■ in special circumstances, under careful medical supervision, nutritionally balanced, very low calorie diets or total fasting for short periods (7–10 days) for rapid weight loss can be effective.

With all of these methods, the major problem in weight reduction is not inducing the initial period of weight loss but, rather, weight regain or recidivism.

Very low calorie diets usually consist of liquid formula meals and should not be utilized unless they contain adequate amounts of high-quality protein (a minimum of 50–60 grams per day) and some carbohydrate (at least 30 grams per day) and are supplemented with vitamins and micronutrients. Patients with type II diabetes who are on such diets should be closely supervised by a physician.

For patients with pronounced fasting hyperglycemia, very low calorie diets (600 kcal/day) are often useful in achieving rapid glycemic control as well as an initial rapid rate of weight loss, which can often be of important psychological and motivational benefit.

Distribution of Calories. In addition to total caloric consumption, attention should be paid to the daily distribution of calories. Calories should be spread as evenly as possible throughout the major daily meals to avoid a large concentration of calories at any one meal, which might overwhelm the diabetic patient's impaired capacity to metabolize foodstuffs. In general, if meals are taken 4 to 5 hours apart, adequate time will be allowed for the postprandial glucose concentration to return to preprandial levels.

For patients receiving exogenous insulin, caloric intake and insulin administration should be temporally adjusted so that adequate calories are consumed to cover periods of peak insulin action. Within this framework, however, flexibility should be allowed so that the patient is not locked into fixed times at which meals and snacks must be consumed on a daily basis. Thus, with proper education, the patient can learn to adjust the time of insulin administration to coincide with the time of day a meal is desired.

Nutrient Content of Diet. Currently, a great deal of attention is being paid to individual foodstuffs in the diabetic diet. When patients consume eucaloric diets, it is important that the diet is properly balanced and nutritionally sound.

Protein. A generally accepted protein requirement is 0.8 g/kg per day for adults, but larger amounts are usually consumed in Western diets. Thus, protein usually accounts for approximately 12 to 20 percent of total caloric consumption. With this as a base, the proportions of fat and carbohydrate are inversely related.

Carbohydrate and Fat. Previous attempts to restrict total carbohydrate content are no longer deemed advisable, and most authorities now advocate liberalization of carbohydrate content to 50 to 60 percent of total calories. This means that total fat intake should not exceed 30 percent. Because diabetic patients are predisposed to macrovascular disease, saturated fat (primarily animal fat) intake should not exceed 10 percent of the total calories. Ideally, cholesterol intake should not exceed 300 milligrams per day.

Carbohydrate Makeup. The makeup of the carbohydrate portion of the diet also requires attention. In the past it was believed that diabetic individuals should rigorously avoid sucrose because it is rapidly absorbed and raises the blood glucose level inordinately. Although this may be true when sucrose is consumed as the sole nutritive component, as in soft drinks or certain candies, it is not as great a problem when modest amounts of sucrose are eaten in a mixed-meal setting. Because of this, up to 5 percent of total carbohydrate intake may be consumed as sucrose, as long as it is taken in the context of a mixed meal and spaced out through the day. This liberalization of attitude about sucrose consumption allows the diabetic patient a wider variety of food choices and, thus, makes the diet more palatable. A side benefit of this approach is improved patient adherence to the dietary prescription and to the other elements of the overall therapeutic plan.

The remainder of the carbohydrate the patient is allowed consists primarily of starches. All complex carbohydrates cannot be lumped together as a single food group, however, because the glycemic response to various starches differs widely; for example, it is lowest for lentils and pasta and highest for bread and potatoes.

Before the precise composition of carbohydrate in the diet can be recommended with certainty, more work is needed to determine the glycemic potency of a large number of foods, singly and together, in diabetic patients. At this stage, it is advisable for the patient to consume 50 to 60 percent of calories as carbohydrate, with modest restriction in sucrose intake and emphasis on ingestion of those complex carbohydrates with low glycemic potency.

Fructose. Fructose is a nutritive sweetener that may have a place in the diabetic diet. This simple carbohydrate is somewhat sweeter than sucrose and has similar properties when prepared in foods. Thus, fructose can be substituted for sucrose in most foods, with little change in taste or texture.

Dietary Fiber. Studies have shown that glycemic excursions are reduced and insulin secretion is diminished when nondiabetic individuals and those with type II diabetes consume high-carbohydrate fiber diets. This beneficial effect is mediated through delayed gastric emptying and overall slowing of the rate of carbohydrate digestion and absorption.

Because large amounts of fiber (10–15 grams per day) are needed to observe these effects, major changes in dietary patterns would be necessary to achieve beneficial results. When consumed as natural foods, there do not seem to be

Table 6. Fiber Content of Selected Foods

FOOD	PORTION SIZE	PLANT FIBER (g)
Breads, Cereals, and Starchy Vegetables (cooked/prepared)		
Beans, kidney	½ cup	**4.5**
Bran (100%), cereal	½ cup	**10.0**
Bread		
Rye	1 slice	**2.7**
White	1 slice	**0.8**
Whole-grain wheat	1 slice	**2.7**
Corn, kernels	⅓ cup	**2.1**
Parsnips	⅔ cup	**5.9**
Peas	½ cup	**5.2**
Potato, white	1 small	**3.8**
Rice, brown	½ cup	**1.3**
Rice, white	½ cup	**0.5**
Squash, winter	½ cup	**3.6**
Sweet potatoes	¼ cup	**2.9**
Fruit (uncooked)		
Apple	1 small	**3.9**
Banana	½ small	**1.3**
Blackberries	½ cup	**3.6**
Grapefruit	½	**1.3**
Orange	1 small	**2.1**
Peach	1 medium	**1.0**
Pineapple	¾ cup	**1.3**
Strawberries	¾ cup	**2.4**
Vegetables (cooked unless indicated by +)		
Asparagus	½ cup	**1.2**
Beans, string	½ cup	**1.7**
Beets	½ cup	**1.5**
Broccoli	½ cup	**2.6**
Carrots	½ cup	**2.2**
Cauliflower	½ cup	**0.9**
Cucumbers +	½ cup	**0.8**
Lettuce +	½ cup	**0.5**
Squash, summer	½ cup	**2.3**
Turnips	½ cup	**1.3**

Anderson, JW, Ward K: Long-term effects of high-carbohydrate, high-fiber diets on glucose and lipid metabolism: a preliminary report on patients with diabetes. *Diabetes Care* 1:77–82, 1978

any untoward effects of increased fiber ingestion, and some studies indicate that increased fiber intake can lower serum triglyceride levels. In obese type II patients, a high-fiber diet may also enhance satiety, which is helpful in maintenance of weight reduction.

Current research is aimed at determining the side effects of high-fiber diets as well as the proper amounts and types of fiber that are most beneficial. Until all the facts are known, it is appropriate to recommend that patients select food containing unrefined carbohydrate with high fiber content rather than highly re-fined carbohydrate with lower fiber content (e.g., an orange rather than orange juice). The fiber content of selected foods is given in Table 6.

Diabetic Complications and Diet
Patients with diabetes mellitus have a greater than normal prevalence of hyperlipidemia, atherosclerosis, and hypertension. In patients with hyper-cholesterolemia, the cholesterol content of the diet should be reduced to less than 300 milligrams per day, and saturated fat should be restricted in favor of polyunsaturated fats. When hypertri-

glyceridemia exists, dietary therapy should consist of weight reduction (if the patient is obese), decreased fat intake, increased polyunsaturated-to-saturated fat ratio, a reduction in simple carbohydrate-containing foods, and marked restriction in alcohol consumption. If hypertension exists, a reduced sodium intake should be encouraged.

Other Food Considerations
When the meal plan is prescribed for a diabetic patient, consideration must also be given to the use of alcoholic beverages and substitute nonnutritive sweeteners.

Alcohol. Strict abstinence from alcohol is not necessary for patients with diabetes mellitus, although alcoholic beverages do add calories without nutritional benefit. In most cases, moderate amounts of alcohol may be allowed. When alcohol is part of the meal plan, it is convenient to account for the calories by reducing the patient's fat intake.

Before a patient may include alcohol in his/her eating plan, the potential problems associated with alcohol consumption should be considered; e.g., excessive alcohol consumption by a person who is fasting or undernourished may lead to hypoglycemia, and this can be a serious problem in patients taking insulin or an oral hypoglycemic agent. Obviously, a patient's ability to follow the prescribed management plan will be impaired if he/she is intoxicated. Finally, alcohol ingestion may be associated with significant elevations in fasting and postprandial plasma triglyceride levels. Because of the increased risk of cardiovascular disease in diabetes, alcohol consumption should probably be avoided if the patient has concomitant hypertriglyceridemia.

Nonnutritive Sweeteners. Because cyclamates have been banned in the United States, saccharin is the only true nonnutritive sweetener available in this country. However, some people find that saccharin has a bitter aftertaste. Aspartame, an amino acid sweetener, is so sweet that it can be considered a nonnutritive sweetener because only minute amounts are used in food products. Aspartame has excellent taste qualities, although it cannot be used in all applications because it loses sweetness when heated. The use of a variety of different sweeteners may be the best op-

tion, maximizing the positive aspects of each. Table 7 presents some characteristics of these sweeteners.

Implementation of Dietary Therapy
Initiation of a specific meal plan requires patient education and often behavior modification. The patient must be taught the principles of good nutrition and learn how to put these principles into effect in a coordinated dietary program geared to the patient's individual requirements.

For the most part, the busy practitioner can only perform the initial examination, obtain a brief diet history, and outline the overall nutritional plan for the patient. In this case, a qualified dietitian or nutritionist assumes responsibility for obtaining the complete dietary history, initiating and prescribing the specific meal plan, and helping the patient to execute it.

For example, it is important to learn all the foods a patient consumes during a typical 24-hour period as well as the circumstances of food consumption (time of day, duration of eating periods, place, simultaneous activities, and emotional state). Much of this information will be used to devise techniques for helping the patient adhere to a specific dietary plan.

Despite the importance of dietary therapy in diabetes, a minority of diabetic patients adhere to the recommended dietary regimen. To a large extent, this failure of dietary therapy is due to inadequate understanding of dietary goals and methods on the part of the patient as well as the physician. An additional factor is that dietary therapy must be individualized, taking into account each patient's life-style, economic status, food preferences, and social needs. One cannot simply provide pamphlets, instructional aids, and meal plans and expect even motivated patients to adhere to the necessary regimen. Detailed instruction by a nutrition counselor is necessary to tailor the diet to each patient's special needs.

Because dietary therapy is a chronic treatment modality, the longer view must be taken when the patient is approached regarding this form of treatment. That is, occasional deviations from recommended meal plans for special occasions are acceptable provided that the patient has a clear understanding of how this should be managed.

Table 7. Alternative Tabletop Sweeteners

For comparison, sucrose (table sugar) contains 16 calories per teaspoon.

SWEETENING AGENT	SOME PRODUCTS AVAILABLE	SWEETNESS EQUIVALENT (Compared with table sugar)	CALORIES	COMMENTS
Aspartame	Equal			Excellent for many uses but undesirable in cooking because, under prolonged heating, sweetness disappears.
	1 packet*	2 tsp.	4	
	1 tablet†	1 tsp.	0.04	
Fructose	Estee Fructose			Occurs naturally in fruits and honey; sweetest when used in cold liquids like lemonade and iced tea.
	1 tsp.	1½ tsp.	16	
Saccharin	Necta Sweet			No calories or carbohydrate; some find aftertaste unpleasant.
	¼-grain tablet	1 tsp.	0	
	½-grain tablet	2 tsp.	0	
	1-grain tablet	4 tsp.	0	
	Sucaryl (liquid)			
	6 drops	1 tsp.	0	
	2 tbsp.	1 cup	0	
	Sweeta			
	2 drops	1 tsp.	0	
	1 tablet	1 tsp.	0	
	Sweet 'N Low			
	(liquid)	1 tsp.		
	10 drops	½ cup	0	
	1 tbsp.		0	
	Sweet 10	1 tsp.		
	(liquid)	½ cup		
	⅛ tsp.		0	
	1 tbsp.		0	
Saccharin (with buffer)	‡Sprinkle Sweet			For some, buffers may remove saccharin's aftertaste, but their calories can add up when used in large quantities.
	1 tsp.	1 tsp.	2	
	‡Sugar Twin			
	1 tsp.	1 tsp.	1½	
	1 packet*	2 tsp.	4	
	*Sweet 'N Low			
	¹⁄₁₀ tsp.	1 tsp.	2	
	1 tsp.	¼ cup	18	
	1 packet	2 tsp.	3½	
	*Sweet 'N Low Brown			
	¹⁄₁₀ tsp.	1 tsp.	2	
	1 tsp.	¼ cup	18	
	*Weight Watchers Sweet'ner			
	⅛ tsp.	1 tsp.	3½	
	1 packet	1 tsp.	3½	

*Packaged with dextrose buffer. †Packaged with lactose buffer. ‡Packaged with dextrin buffer.
Adapted from Crapo P: A survey of sweeteners (Abstract). *Clin Diabetes* 1:21, 1983

Table 8. Major Deterrents to Successful Diet Therapy

Diabetic patients on a strict diet should take precaution against the following:

- failure to understand that elevated blood glucose levels are frequently associated with obesity and that attainment and maintenance of desirable body weight is one main and profoundly beneficial objective in treatment of type II diabetes mellitus;
- failure to determine appropriate diet prescription;
- failure to use appropriately trained dietitians for counseling;
- using old, incomplete, or inappropriate diet materials for individual needs;
- failure to adapt diet to individual's life-style and other needs;
- failure to change patient's behavior because of inadequate education or follow-up care;
- failure to understand magnitude and number of obstacles to be overcome in achieving results;
- failure to adapt teaching techniques to individual;
- confusion about dietary goals, strategies, and priorities for individual patients;
- uncertainty about influence of diet on blood glucose and lipid levels; and
- limited educational programs because of economic factors, including lack of third-party coverage for good counseling programs.

Adapted from Davidson JK: A new look at diet therapy. *Diabetes Forecast* May/June:14–19, 1976

Often, a little leeway allows for better patient compliance with the overall diet plan. Periodic meetings with a nutrition counselor are necessary to implement and maintain individualized dietary regimens.

The common reasons for failure of dietary therapy are listed in Table 8. Keeping these reasons in mind and taking remedial action as necessary will help the clinician and the patient succeed with the most important part of the therapeutic plan for this disease (see Helping Patient Cope).

Appropriate Physical Activity

The typical patient with type II diabetes mellitus is a good candidate for an exercise program. Obesity and inactivity contribute to the development of glucose intolerance in this genetically predisposed individual, and regular exercise has a positive influence on the major pathogenic mechanisms in this disease. Exercise also has a positive influence on certain cardiovascular risk factors, which worsen the prognosis in

these patients. In addition, a review of pertinent literature on the effects of exercise in patients with type II diabetes leads to the conclusion that the potential and actual benefits of regular exercise far outweigh the potential and actual risks.

Although it appears sensible to make exercise a part of the treatment plan for a patient with type II diabetes mellitus, it should be emphasized that more research is needed in this area and that the actual benefits, risks, and guidelines for prescribing exercise are not yet precisely defined.

Actual and Potential Benefits of Exercise

If certain precautions are observed, increased physical activity has several actual and potential benefits to offer the patient with type II diabetes mellitus. The benefits of this enjoyable and inexpensive therapy include the following:
- improvement in insulin sensitivity and potential improvement in glucose tolerance in some individuals;
- adjunct to diet in the promotion of weight loss and maintenance of ideal body weight;
- amelioration of cardiovascular risk factors;
- potential reduction in dosage or need for insulin or oral hypoglycemic agents;
- enhancement of work capacity; and
- enrichment of quality of life and improvement in sense of well-being.

Improvement in Insulin Sensitivity/Glucose Tolerance. It is well known that glucose tolerance is impaired by prolonged physical inactivity (e.g., many days of bed rest). It is also known from a number of studies, beginning in the early 1970s, that obesity-associated peripheral resistance to insulin can be reversed or improved with physical activity and that this exercise-induced enhanced sensitivity to insulin occurs without changes in body weight. Other studies indicate that improvements in glucose tolerance due to physical training in obese individuals with type II diabetes mellitus are modest at best and do not persist when training is discontinued. In such individuals, there is a small but significant increase in sensitivity to insulin when a physical training program is added to weight reduction by dieting. Moderate intensity exercise usually has a blood glucose lowering effect in people with type II diabetes, which may persist for several hours after completion of the exercise. Because of this, repeated bouts of exercise may, over time, result in lower mean blood glucose concentrations and improved metabolic control, as measured by glycohemoglobin concentrations.

Even though the benefit is not large, the data favor the prescription of an appropriate increase in physical activity, especially for the obese patient who is engaged in a weight-reduction program.

Adjunct to Diet in Promotion of Weight Loss/Maintenance of Ideal Body Weight. Increased physical activity is recognized as an important part of weight-reduction programs because it increases energy expenditure and may help to motivate the patient to increase weight reduction efforts. Under relatively sedentary weight-stable conditions, energy expenditure through physical activity accounts for approximately 20 percent of total daily caloric requirements. Addition of an exercise program can increase this to 35 or 40 percent of total daily energy expenditure. Physical exercise alone usually does not result in significant weight loss but may alter body composition by increasing muscle mass and decreasing body fat. When combined with caloric restriction, exercise is an excellent way to increase negative caloric balance. Under these conditions, low-calorie diets should contain enough carbohydrate to maintain adequate muscle glycogen stores if high-intensity exercise is anticipated.

Cardiovascular Benefits. The value of physical training in ameliorating risk factors for cardiovascular disease has been amply demonstrated in nondiabetic individuals. Exercise is associated with a reduction in circulating levels of very-low-density lipoprotein and low-density lipoprotein (LDL) cholesterol, triglycerides, and insulin. In addition to the known coronary risk of elevated LDL cholesterol and triglycerides, serum insulin levels have been shown to have a direct correlation with coronary risk as well. Exercise also is associated with increases in high-density lipoprotein cholesterol, which may protect against cardiovascular disease. Furthermore, exercise is associated with decreases in blood pressure and cardiac work both at rest and during exercise as well as increases in maximum oxygen uptake and total working capacity.

The beneficial effects of exercise on risk factors in patients with type II diabetes mellitus have not been extensively studied, but it is reasonable to assume that exercise might help to prevent or retard cardiovascular complications in this particularly susceptible group of individuals. Again, however, the cardiovascular and metabolic benefits of exercise are not sustained when training is discontinued.

Other Benefits. Increased work capacity, potential reduction in dosage or need for pharmacologic intervention to achieve metabolic control, and improvement in sense of well-being are among the other possible benefits of an exercise program.

Actual and Potential Risks of Exercise

Adverse metabolic and hormonal side effects as a consequence of physical exercise are rarely reported in patients with type II diabetes mellitus. There are potential hazards, however.

Prolonged and vigorous exercise can potentiate the hypoglycemic effects of both oral agents and insulin. Hypoglycemia during or after exercise is a definite risk in a patient taking insulin. If insulin deficiency is severe and the patient is poorly controlled (blood glucose >300 mg/dl), exercise may cause deterioration of metabolic control.

Because accelerated atherosclerotic heart disease is common in patients with type II diabetes, there is a risk that exercise will precipitate arrhythmia and myocardial ischemia or infarction. In the obese patient, degenerative joint disease may be aggravated by certain types of exercise, and ligamentous injuries are more common.

The potential hazards of exercise can be prevented or reduced if the program is preceded by a thorough medical evaluation and is planned to start with relatively low levels of physical exertion, progressing gradually to higher levels of work. The patient should be well informed about the benefits and risks of exercise, and supervision is highly desirable, at least initially. The principles governing exercise in a patient with diabetes are the same as those used in cardiac rehabilitation programs. In fact, it might be wise to involve patients with known atherosclerotic disease in a cardiac rehabilitation or similarly structured and supervised program rather than to assume responsibility for this aspect of treatment.

Indications and Contraindications
Unless contraindicated, appropriate physical activity should be recommended as an adjunct to proper nutrition for patients with type II diabetes mellitus. Exercise should be prescribed with caution if the patient
■ has poorly controlled labile blood glucose levels;
■ is at increased risk because of diabetic complications including significant atherosclerosis, proliferative retinopathy, or neuropathy; or
■ is unable to prevent hypoglycemia induced by prolonged and vigorous exercise.

Guidelines for Exercise Prescription
The key to a successful exercise program is individualization. The exercise program must be designed with the particular patient in mind and take into account the interests, initial physical condition, and motivation of the patient (see Helping the Patient Cope).

A safe and logical exercise prescription is based on a complete medical evaluation and requires that special instructions be given to the patient for managing the exercise program. The patient should start slowly, exercise at regular intervals at least three or four times weekly, and gradually increase the duration and intensity of the exercise to achieve and maintain a training effect (see Guidelines for the Exercise Prescription, below). Most patients can at least undertake a walking program, which is relatively safe.

Guidelines for the Exercise Prescription

The following guidelines should be observed when advising or prescribing an exercise program for a patient with type II diabetes mellitus.

Perform a detailed medical evaluation of the patient before initiating an exercise program.
This medical evaluation should include the following:
■ determination of glycemic control;
■ cardiovascular examination (blood pressure, peripheral pulses, bruits, blood lipids, ECG at rest and during exercise if the patient is over 40 years old or has a history of cardiovascular disease);
■ determination of working capacity (graduated exercise test with measurement of pulse rate response or oxygen consumption);
■ chest roentgenogram;
■ neurologic examination;
■ ophthalmoscopic examination; and
■ detailed ophthalmologic evaluation if proliferative retinopathy is present or suspected.

Strenuous exercise is contraindicated for patients with poor metabolic control and for those with significant diabetic complications (particularly, active proliferative retinopathy, significant cardiovascular disease, and neuropathy).

Special precautions should be taken when the patient requires or uses drugs that may make him/her more susceptible to exercise-induced hypoglycemia. For example, alcohol and very high doses of salicylates should be avoided because they may, by themselves, produce hypoglycemia. The beta-adrenergic blocking agents may prevent the rapid hepatic glycogenolytic responses that normally correct hypoglycemia. Certain other drugs, including bishydroxycoumarin, phenylbutazone, sulfonamides, and monoamine oxidase inhibitors, may potentiate the action of sulfonylurea agents.

Prescribe a program of exercise tailored to the patient's physical capacity and interests.
The program should always start with low work loads (see Table 9), gradually increase to higher work loads, and be supervised, at least initially.

Each exercise session should include appropriate warm-up and cool-down periods. Most programs include a combination of stretching and flexibility exercises, strength-building exercises, and aerobic endurance exercises. In general, the best cardiovascular benefits will be observed with a graduated program that emphasizes aerobic endurance exercises.

An appropriate plan is to start each exercise session with 5 to 10 minutes of stretching and flexibility exercises followed by 20 to 30 minutes of strenuous exercises of sufficient intensity to sustain the pulse rate at approximately 75 percent of the maximal heart rate response (resting pulse plus 0.75 times the difference between maximum pulse rate and resting pulse rate). During training, the work required to maintain the submaximal pulse rate will gradually increase. The exercise session should conclude with 15 to 20 minutes of less-strenuous exercise and stretching to provide a cooling-down period. During training, at least three or four sessions per week are recommended until the desired fitness level is achieved. Once the desired level of training is achieved, fitness can usually be maintained by three exercise sessions per week.

Patients with insensitive feet should avoid exercises that involve running, because running is potentially traumatizing; cycling and swimming are good alternatives.

Patients who select running or jogging should have a careful evaluation of their feet by a qualified health-care professional before initiation of their exercise program. They also need instruction on how to select protective footwear.

Patients with active proliferative retinopathy should avoid strenuous, high-intensity exercises associated with Valsalva-like maneuvers, such as weight lifting and certain types of isometrics. These patients should also avoid head-low positions such as might occur with yoga. They should not participate in activities associated with excessive jarring and jolting of the head.

Patients with hypertension should avoid heavy lifting, straining, and Valsalva-like maneuvers, which raise blood pressure. They should also avoid intense exercises involving the arms and upper body, which cause greater increases in blood pressure than exercises involving major muscle groups of the lower extremities. Rhythmic exercises involving the lower extremities, such as walking, jogging, and cycling, are generally preferred for patients with hypertension.

Give all patients instructions for safe participation in exercise programs. Tell patients to do the following:
■ carry a card or wear a bracelet at all times that identifies them as having diabetes mellitus;
■ be alert for the signs and symptoms of hypoglycemia during and up to several hours after exercise;
■ have a source of readily absorbable carbohydrate available during exercise that can

be used to prevent or treat hypoglycemia; and
■ avoid the risk of dehydration (which may be a problem when metabolic control is less than desired) by taking extra fluids or by skipping exercise on particularly warm days.

Special Instructions for well-controlled insulin-taking diabetic patients who plan to participate in strenuous exercise

Individuals taking insulin vary considerably in their responses to exercise. Therefore, it may be helpful to monitor blood glucose concentrations closely from time to time to determine the response to the type, intensity, and duration of exercise being performed. The information gained from such monitoring can be used to individualize the adjustments in insulin and diet that must be made to maintain good control and to avoid hypoglycemia during or after exercise. The following instructions are useful starting points.
■ Choose a time to exercise when the blood sugar level is above fasting values, perhaps 1 to 3 hours after a meal.
■ To avoid hypoglycemia, it may be necessary to consume extra carbohydrate before, during, and after exercise.
■ If the diabetes is well controlled with a single daily dose of intermediate-acting insulin, decrease the dose on days when exercise is planned. Some patients will require a decrease in insulin dosage of as much as 30 to 35 percent or a shift to a schedule of two or more doses per day, with or without the addition of short-acting insulin.
■ If using a combination of intermediate- and short-acting insulin, decrease or omit the short-acting insulin dose and decrease the dose of intermediate-acting insulin by up to one-third. Under these circumstances, hyperglycemia may occur later in the day and require a second injection of short-acting insulin.
■ If using only short-acting insulin, the dose before exercise should be reduced appropriately, and postexercise doses should be adjusted (usually reduced) based on glucose monitoring and experience with postexercise hypoglycemia. Some patients require a dosage reduction of as much as 30 to 50 percent.

Reevaluate the patient after 6 months, after 12 months, and then yearly.

Table 9. Energy Expenditure Associated With Common Exercises

ACTIVITY	CALORIES BURNED (min)	CALORIES BURNED (hr)
Light housework Polishing furniture Light washing by hand	2–2½	120–150
Golf, using power cart Level walking at 2 miles per hour	2½–4	150–240
Cleaning windows, mopping floors, or vacuuming Walking at 3 miles per hour Golf, pulling cart Cycling at 6 miles per hour Bowling	4–5	240–300
Scrubbing floors Cycling 8 miles per hour Walking 3½ miles per hour Table tennis, badminton, and volleyball Doubles tennis Golf, carrying clubs Many calisthenics and ballet exercises	5–6	300–360
Walking 4 miles per hour Ice or roller skating Cycling 10 miles per hour	6–7	360–420
Walking 5 miles per hour Cycling 11 miles per hour Water skiing Singles tennis	7–8	420–480
Jogging 5 miles per hour Cycling 12 miles per hour Downhill skiing Paddleball	8–10	480–600
Running 5½ miles per hour Cycling 13 miles per hour Squash or handball (practice session)	10–11	600–660
Running 6 miles per hour or more Competitive handball or squash	11 or more	660 or more

Adapted from Rifkin H (Ed.): *The American Diabetes Association Guide to Good Living.* New York, American Diabetes Association, 1982

Summary

Current evidence suggests that improvement in insulin sensitivity and some reduction in cardiovascular risk factors can be achieved with relatively mild training. Consequently, appropriate increases in physical activity can be planned for all patients in whom exercise is not contraindicated. For some patients, appropriate physical activity will involve strenuous and formalized physical training. For other patients, it will mean taking the stairs instead of taking the elevator. Clearly, however, increased physical activity is an adjunct to rather than a substitute for attention to proper nutrition and weight reduction.

Pharmacologic Intervention

Pharmacologic intervention should be considered when the patient with type II diabetes cannot achieve normal or near-normal plasma glucose levels with dietary modification and regular exercise. The two options for this stage of therapy are oral hypoglycemic agents and insulin.

The question is: Which pharmacologic alternative is best for the patient? The practicing physician can determine the answer to that question, in part, by considering the following:
- the severity of the patient's disease (i.e., degree of hyperglycemia, presence/absence of symptoms);
- the condition of the patient otherwise (presence/absence of concurrent diseases and conditions);
- the preferences of the patient who has been well informed about the use, expected therapeutic effects, and possible side effects of oral agents and insulin;
- the motivation of the patient; and
- age and weight of the patient.

Major concerns about the safety of oral hypoglycemic agents, which were raised in 1970 when the University Group Diabetes Program (UGDP) study was published, have diminished because there is no agreement on interpretation of data from that study. Furthermore, problems with study design make a valid interpretation of the UGDP data somewhat difficult.

The major benefit of the UGDP study was to focus attention on treatment of type II diabetes in general and on the use of oral hypoglycemic agents in particular. As a result of the study, most clinicians agree that the cornerstone of therapy for type II diabetes is dietary modification plus regular exercise and that the use of any pharmacologic agent is an adjunct to rather than a substitute for dietary modification and exercise.

Overview of Treatment With Oral Hypoglycemic Agents

Oral hypoglycemic agents are often therapeutically effective in patients with type II diabetes, and many of these patients are treated with this modality. The mechanism of action of sulfonylurea agents is complex. Acutely, they augment beta-cell insulin secretion. After several months of therapy, however, insulin levels return to pretreatment values, whereas glucose levels remain improved. These findings have led to the suggestion that sulfonylurea drugs exert extrapancreatic effects on glucose metabolism. A number of such effects have been clearly defined. Sulfonylurea compounds reduce the accelerated rates of hepatic glucose production in type II diabetes, partially reverse the postreceptor defect in insulin action, and lead to an increase in the number of cellular insulin receptors. The relative importance of each of these actions in ameliorating hyperglycemia is unclear, but it is likely that pancreatic and extrapancreatic effects of these agents combine to produce the hypoglycemic action of these drugs.

The use of an oral hypoglycemic agent should be seriously considered only if it is clear that there are no contraindications to its use. For example, oral hypoglycemic agents require the presence of endogenous insulin and, therefore, are ineffective and contraindicated for patients with type I diabetes mellitus. In addition, oral agents should not be used during pregnancy and lactation because the effects of oral agents on the fetus and/or newborn are unknown, and oral agents are unlikely to provide adequate glycemic control during stress-producing gestation and lactation. Similarly, oral hypoglycemic agents are not recommended for the treatment of patients with particularly stressful concurrent diseases or conditions, including infection, trauma, acute myocardial infarction, and so on. Finally, oral hypoglycemic agents are contraindicated in patients who are known to be allergic to sulfonylurea compounds.

Having excluded patients with contraindications to oral agents, it is useful to consider the factors that predispose to favorable therapeutic responses to these drugs. The patient most likely to respond well to sulfonylurea drugs is one who
- has had the onset of diabetes after 40 years of age;
- has had diabetes for fewer than 5 years;
- is normal weight or obese;
- has never received insulin or has been well controlled on less than 40 units per day.

Clinical Use of Oral Hypoglycemic Agents

The sulfonylurea agents are the only available oral hypoglycemic agents in the United States that have been approved by the Food and Drug Administration. To use these agents most appropriately, it is useful to consider them in terms of potency, pharmacokinetics, and metabolism, as well as possible complications, factors that influence choice of agents, guidelines for prescription, and possible reasons for drug failure.

Potency, Pharmacokinetics, and Metabolism. There are several different kinds of sulfonylurea compounds, which differ primarily in terms of potency, pharmacokinetics, and modes of metabolism, as outlined in Table 10.

Tolbutamide (Orinase). Tolbutamide is a short-acting sulfonylurea drug that is usually taken two or three times a day. This drug is metabolized by the liver to a totally inactive product that is excreted in the urine. On a weight basis, tolbutamide is the least potent of the available sulfonylurea agents, and some consider this drug safer than other agents, particularly for patients with renal impairment.

Chlorpropamide (Diabinese). Chlorpropamide is partially metabolized by the liver to metabolites that retain hypoglycemic activity, and these metabolites plus intact drug are excreted in the urine. Chlorpropamide has the longest duration of action (~60 hours) and is only given once per day. This compound can cause significant water retention and hyponatremia, primarily by potentiating antidiuretic hormone (ADH) action on the kidney. In addition, the Antabuse-like reaction (alcohol flushing) is seen most commonly with this agent.

Tolazamide (Tolinase). Tolazamide is an intermediate-duration sulfonylurea compound that is metabolized by the liver. The by-products of metabolism have relatively little hypoglycemic activity and are excreted in the urine. Tola-

---

Table 10. Characteristics of Sulfonylurea Agents

GENERIC NAME	BRAND NAME	DAILY DOSAGE RANGE (mg)	DURATION OF ACTION (hr)	COMMENTS
Tolbutamide	Orinase Generic	500–3,000	6–12	Metabolized by liver to an inactive product; given 2 to 3 times per day
Chlorpropamide	Diabinese Generic	100–500	60	Metabolized by liver (~70 percent) to less-active metabolites and excreted intact (~30 percent) by kidneys; can potentiate ADH action; given once per day
Acetohexamide	Dymelor	250–1,500	12–18	Metabolized by liver to active metabolite; given 1 to 2 times per day
Tolazamide	Tolinase Generic	100–1,000	12–24	Metabolized by liver to both active and inactive products; given 1 to 2 times per day
Glipizide	Glucatrol	5–40	12–24	Metabolized by liver to inert products; given 1 to 2 times per day
Glyburide	Diabeta Micronase	2.5–20	16–24	Metabolized by liver to mostly inert products; given 1 to 2 times per day

zamide, which is usually taken once or twice a day, also has diuretic activity.

Acetohexamide (Dymelor). This intermediate-duration sulfonylurea drug, which is taken once or twice a day, is metabolized by the liver to an active metabolite that has more than twice the potency of the original compound. Acetohexamide has diuretic activity and also is a potent uricosuric agent.

Glipizide (Glucatrol). This so-called second-generation sulfonylurea is of intermediate duration. It is taken once or twice a day and has a duration of action of 12 to 24 hours. It is metabolized by the liver to inactive products that are excreted in the urine, and to a lesser extent, in the bile. It is as efficacious as chlorpropamide and has a low incidence of side effects.

Glyburide (Diabeta and Micronase). This so-called second-generation sulfonylurea has a duration of action of 16 to 24 hours. It can be given once or twice a day. It is metabolized by the liver to several weakly active and inactive derivatives. It is excreted in the urine and the bile. It is as efficacious as chlorpropamide. Its profile of side effects is low.

Complications of Sulfonylurea Therapy. Severe hypoglycemia is the major complication of sulfonylurea therapy and has been a particular problem with chlorpropamide because of its long duration of action. Elderly patients are more susceptible to hypoglycemia, particularly when they have a tendency to skip meals or when liver, renal, or cardiovascular function is impaired.

Other side effects of sulfonylurea agents include hematologic reactions (leukopenia, thrombocytopenia, hemolytic anemia), skin reactions (e.g., rashes, purpura, pruritus), antithyroid activity, and diffuse pulmonary reactions. The gastrointestinal effects include nausea, vomiting, and cholestasis (with and without jaundice). Cholestatic jaundice has been identified more often with the use of chlorpropamide than with any other oral agent. Renal side effects include mild diuresis seen with the use of tolazamide and acetohexamide, as well as significant fluid retention and hyponatremia seen with chlorpropamide. The latter effect occurs chiefly because chlorpropamide potentiates the action of ADH on distal renal tubular cells.

In addition to the uncommon side effects cited above, there are many drugs that can potentiate or interfere with the hypoglycemic action of sulfonylurea drugs. Table 28 lists some of the most important of these drugs, and their administration with sulfonylureas must be carefully monitored.

Choice of Agent. The initial choice of an oral hypoglycemic drug depends on the patient's nutritional intake and physical condition. For example, patients who skip meals are particularly susceptible to hypoglycemia. Patients with impaired renal function are particularly susceptible to hypoglycemia caused by chlorpropamide because of its long action and by acetohexamide because of its very active metabolite. Patients with cardiovascular disease such as hypertension and congestive heart failure may experience adverse effects with the use of chlorpropamide because of its ADH-potentiating activity. In general, older patients have more renal failure and cardiovascular and hepatic problems, as well as a tendency to skip meals and snacks. For this reason, it is best to choose an agent with relatively short duration of action, which is less likely to cause profound hypoglycemia.

Drug Administration. After the most appropriate agent is selected for a particular patient, the lowest effective dose should be prescribed. The dose should be increased every 1 or 2 weeks until satisfactory glycemic control or the maximum dose is reached. If the maximum dose of the initially selected agent does not provide adequate glycemic control, then it is common practice to try another oral agent. If control is not achieved after two oral agents, the patient is a candidate for insulin therapy. No benefit is achieved by using two sulfonylurea drugs simultaneously.

Drug Failures. Approximately 60 to 70 percent of patients with type II diabetes will demonstrate an initial satisfactory response to sulfonylurea therapy. When a patient does not respond initially, this is called primary failure. When initial glycemic control is achieved with an oral agent and then lost, the patient is considered a secondary drug failure. Secondary drug failure occurs in 5 to 10 percent of patients per year, depending on the characteristics of the population studied. In some cases, secondary failure occurs because the patient does not follow the prescribed diet, and correction of dietary indiscretion can restore the desired glycemic effect of the drug. In other cases of secondary failure, progression of disease should be considered, as should the occurrence of an underlying stressful disease or condition such as infection, pregnancy, or cardiovascular disease. In these situations, the patient should be switched to insulin. After recovery from an intercurrent disease or condition, reinstitution of oral hypoglycemic therapy may be successful.

Overview of Insulin Therapy

Insulin is capable of restoring glycemia to normal in most patients with type II diabetes, and many physicians prefer it to oral hypoglycemic agents as the primary pharmacologic intervention (i.e., after diet and exercise have failed to normalize blood glucose). There are several additional circumstances that are absolute indications for the use of insulin. These circumstances include the following:
■ periods of acute injury, stress, infection, or surgery (in such circumstances, insulin requirements are increased, and dietary management with or without a concomitant oral hypoglycemic agent is inadequate);
■ pregnancy; and
■ allergy or serious reaction to sulfonylurea drugs.

Note that any metabolic state or drug that increases requirements for insulin or interferes with insulin secretion will, in all probability, convert the non-insulin-dependent patient with type II diabetes into an insulin-requiring patient. (Management of patients with insulin during pregnancy and surgery is discussed on pages 45–47.)

Insulin lowers the blood glucose by increasing glucose uptake and metabolism by insulin-sensitive peripheral tissues (such as muscle and adipose tissue) and by suppressing hepatic glucose production. It also promotes the storage of energy in the form of adipose tissue triglycerides.

Because patients with type II diabetes are resistant to insulin action, one might presume that they would require large doses of insulin to normalize their blood glucose. Obesity is another cause of resistance to insulin action. Thus, obese type II diabetic patients (which account for ~75 percent of all type II patients) should be particularly difficult to control on insulin and might be expected to require very large quantities of insulin given more than once a day as a mixture of short- and intermediate-acting insulins to achieve control.

Indeed, many experienced clinicians have the impression that insulin treatment of patients with type II diabetes is generally disappointing. These clinicians acknowledge that insulin therapy initially decreases the blood glucose toward normal. They point out, however, that the patient treated with insulin frequently has an increased appetite, eats more, gains weight, becomes more insulin resistant, experiences increases in fasting glucose levels, and then requires even more insulin. Note that there are no adequately controlled studies to validate this clinical impression.

Clinical Use of Insulin

Clinical experience with insulin therapy for patients with type II diabetes depends on the characteristics of the patient population under study. A few studies involving small numbers of relatively nonobese patients who have had type II diabetes for several years and moderate to severe fasting hyperglycemia (~250 mg/dl) suggest that these patients are quite resistant to insulin action and require doses of insulin in excess of 100 units per day as well as intensive treatment (2 or more injections of mixtures of insulins per day) to control their hyperglycemia.

On the other hand, several large, well-controlled studies suggest that modest doses of insulin and relatively simple treatment programs can achieve good metabolic regulation in some newly diagnosed, generally obese patients with mild to moderately severe type II diabetes. Of note are the UGDP study and a study from Great Britain that is currently underway.

The UGDP study was a multicenter collaborative study of the treatment of patients with mild to moderately severe type II diabetes over a period of 10 years. As one facet of its investigation, the UGDP compared the regulation of fasting and postprandial blood glucose levels by variable insulin treatment with that by placebo and diet. Placebo and diet treatment for 10 years resulted in a significant rise in plasma glucose (22 percent above baseline values), whereas appropriate insulin treatment for 10 years resulted in maintaining the fasting plasma glucose 20 percent lower than the initial baseline values. As noted in Table 11, most patients initially maintained a fasting plasma glucose of about 120 mg/dl on less than 20 units of insulin given once a day. In contrast, by 10 years, 44 percent of patients required 40 or more units of insulin per day. The mean insulin requirement for all patients rose approximately fivefold over the 10 years.

The complications of insulin therapy in the UGDP study were not striking. Forty-one percent of the patients had to have a single adjustment of insulin management because of presumed hypoglycemia, and 25 percent had two or more adjustments. Patients on insulin management maintained their obesity but did not become more obese, whereas patients in the diet and placebo group lost about 5 percent of their body weight over the 10-year period.

The results of the multicenter study in Great Britain are similar to the UGDP study. After 1 year of treatment, type II patients initially requiring insulin treatment were taking an average of 31 units of insulin per day with 50 percent of the patients on single and the other 50 percent on multiple injections per day. The insulin-treated patients gained 2 kilograms of body weight in the 1st year.

Several points about insulin therapy can be drawn from clinical studies.
■ Insulin treatment can be used to achieve euglycemia in patients with type II diabetes mellitus.
■ Newly diagnosed patients with mild to moderately severe fasting hyperglycemia can be controlled with modest doses of insulin given once or several times a day.
■ With time, insulin requirements should be expected to increase in patients with type II diabetes.
■ Patients with type II diabetes of many years' duration and those with

---

Table 11. Insulin Dose Necessary to Maintain Fasting Plasma Glucose of 120 mg/dl

DOSE (U/Day)	FIRST 3 MONTHS OF TREATMENT (% of Patients)	10TH YEAR OF TREATMENT (% of Patients)
<20	89	37
20–39	9	19
40–59	2	17
60–74		14
75+		13

From University Group Diabetes Program: Effects of hypoglycemic agents on vascular complications in patients with adult-onset diabetes. VIII. Evaluation of insulin therapy: final report. *Diabetes* 31 (Suppl. 5):1–26, 1982

---

moderate to severe hyperglycemia are more resistant to insulin action and may require large doses of insulin to control hyperglycemia.
■ When large doses of insulin are required, it is best to split the dose into two or more injections and to use a combination of short-acting insulin plus intermediate- or long-acting insulin.
■ Although increased appetite and weight gain are potential side effects of insulin treatment, careful dietary management can lessen the impact of these potential problems.

Various Types of Insulin and Their Characteristics. The appropriate use of insulin requires familiarity with the various available types of insulin and some knowledge of their characteristics. Table 12 lists the insulins sold in the United States in 1987. Insulins are classified by types and duration of action.

Types of Insulin. A wide variety of purified insulins are available. Beef insulin is considerably more antigenic than pork or human insulin, so the use of beef insulin alone or in mixtures with pork insulin is associated with more insulin allergy, insulin resistance due to excessive insulin antibodies, and lipoatrophy than is the use of pure pork or human insulin.

The selection of a specific insulin preparation is dictated by the nature of the patient to be treated. Human or pork insulin is certainly indicated for pa-

Table 12. Insulins Sold in the United States

PRODUCT	MANUFACTURER	FORM	STRENGTH
Rapid acting (onset 0.5—4 hr)			
Humulin regular	Lilly	Human	U-100
Humulin BR (for external insulin pumps only)	Lilly	Human	U-100
Novolin R (regular; formerly Actrapid human)	Squibb-Novo	Human	U-100
Velosulin human (regular)	Nordisk-USA	Human	U-100
Iletin II regular	Lilly	Beef	U-100
Iletin II regular	Lilly	Pork	U-100, U-500
Purified pork R (regular; formerly Actrapid)	Squibb-Novo	Pork	U-100
Velosulin (regular)	Nordisk-USA	Pork	U-100
Purified pork S (Semilente; formerly Semitard)	Squibb-Novo	Pork	U-100
Iletin I regular	Lilly	Beef/Pork	U-40, U-100
Regular	Squibb-Novo	Pork	U-100
Iletin I Semilente	Lilly	Beef/Pork	U-40, U-100
Semilente	Squibb-Novo	Beef	U-100
Novolin R Penfill (regular)	Squibb-Novo	Human	U-100
Intermediate acting (onset 1—4 hr)			
Humulin L	Lilly	Human	U-100
Humulin NPH	Lilly	Human	U-100
Insulatard human NPH	Nordisk-USA	Human	U-100
Novolin L (lente; formerly Monotard human)	Squibb-Novo	Human	U-100
Novolin N (NPH)	Squibb-Novo	Human	U-100
Iletin II Lente	Lilly	Beef	U-100
Iletin II NPH	Lilly	Beef	U-100
Iletin II Lente	Lilly	Pork	U-100
Iletin II NPH	Lilly	Pork	U-100
Insulatard NPH	Nordisk-USA	Pork	U-100
Purified pork lente (formerly Monotard)	Squibb-Novo	Pork	U-100
Purified pork N (NPH; formerly Protaphane)	Squibb-Novo	Pork	U-100
Iletin I Lente	Lilly	Beef/Pork	U-40, U-100
Iletin I NPH	Lilly	Beef/Pork	U-40, U-100
NPH	Squibb-Novo	Beef	U-100
Long acting (onset 4—6 hr)			
Iletin II PZI	Lilly	Beef	U-100
Iletin II PZI	Lilly	Pork	U-100
Purified beef U (ultralente; formerly Ultratard)	Squibb-Novo	Beef	U-100
Iletin I PZI	Lilly	Beef/Pork	U-40, U-100
Iletin I Ultralente	Lilly	Beef/Pork	U-40, U-100
Ultralente	Squibb-Novo	Beef	U-100
Humulin U (Ultralente)	Lilly	Human	U-100
Mixtures			
Mixtard (30% regular, 70% NPH)	Nordisk-USA	Pork	U-100
Novolin 70/30	Squibb-Novo	Human	U-100

tients with insulin allergy, severe insulin resistance due to insulin antibodies, or lipoatrophy. Patients who are candidates for intermittent insulin therapy (e.g., those who require insulin because of onset of diabetes during pregnancy or for acute problems such as infection, myocardial infarction, and emergency surgery) also should be treated with human or pork insulin to minimize the likelihood of insulin allergy or the ultimate development of insulin resistance. As the cost of human insulin decreases, this preparation is likely to become the initial choice for all patients with type II diabetes who require insulin therapy.

Duration of Action. The selection of an appropriate insulin preparation also depends on the desired course of action (Table 13). Patients with mild to moderate fasting hyperglycemia may adequately control their condition with one injection of intermediate-acting insulin before breakfast.

Many patients with type II diabetes need an insulin regimen consisting of short-acting insulin with either intermediate-acting or long-acting insulin (Figure 2).

Typical Insulin Program. A typical insulin program might include an injection of a mixture of NPH or lente insulin with regular insulin in the morning, one-half hour before breakfast, and another injection of the same mixture in the evening, one-half hour before the evening meal. The ratio of intermediate-acting insulin to regular insulin in the morning is 2:1 and in the evening 1:1. Adjustments of the dosage and amount of each type of insulin are made to modify the blood glucose level at the appropriate times of the day, as shown in Figure 2. Mixing insulins may alter the peak and duration of action of insulins. This may be a particular problem when mixing regular with lente insulins.

Dosage Requirements. The total dose of insulin needed by a patient with type II diabetes may be as little as 5 to 10 units per day or as much as several hundred units per day. Because insulin resistance is a significant component of both type II diabetes and obesity, it is evident that some obese patients with type II diabetes may require large quantities of insulin ($>$100 units per day) to appropriately control hyperglycemia. When smaller doses of insulin suffice ($<$30 units per day), a single injection of intermediate-acting insulin in the

Table 13. Time Course of Action of Insulin Preparations*

INSULIN PREPARATION	ONSET OF ACTION	PEAK ACTION	DURATION OF ACTION
Short acting			
Regular Iletin II (crystalline-zinc)	15–30 min	2–4 hr	5–7 hr
Novolin R	30 min	2½–5 hr	5–8 hr
Velosulin	30 min	2–5 hr	5–8 hr
Humulin R	30 min	2–4 hr	6–8 hr
Intermediate acting			
Lente	1–2 hr	6–12 hr	18–24 hr
NPH	1–2 hr	6–12 hr	18–24 hr
Novolin L	2½–5 hr	7–15 hr	18–24 hr
Humulin N	1–3 hr	6–12 hr	14–24 hr
Novolin 70/30	30 min	7–12 hr	24 hr
Long acting			
Ultralente (beef/pork)	4–6 hr	14–24 hr	28–36 hr
Humulin U	4–6 hr	8–20 hr	24–28 hr

*Average values. Considerable variation is found in individual diabetic patients.

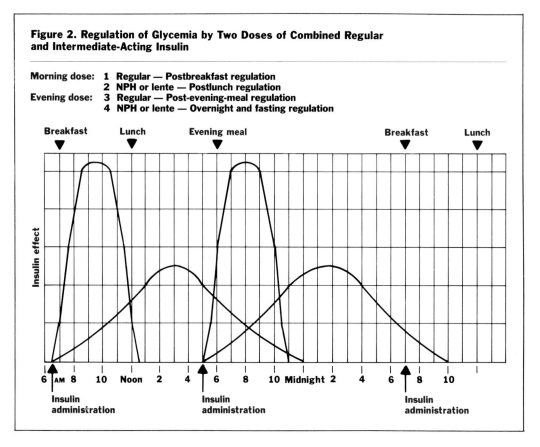

Figure 2. Regulation of Glycemia by Two Doses of Combined Regular and Intermediate-Acting Insulin

Morning dose: 1 Regular — Postbreakfast regulation
2 NPH or lente — Postlunch regulation
Evening dose: 3 Regular — Post-evening-meal regulation
4 NPH or lente — Overnight and fasting regulation

morning may be adequate. When insulin doses above 30 units a day are required, two injections, usually with mixtures of regular and intermediate-acting insulins, are probably preferable.

Complications of Insulin Therapy. The complications of insulin therapy in the patient with type II diabetes, which are the same as those that occur in patients with type I diabetes, include hypoglycemia, lipodystrophies, antibody formation including insulin resistance, and allergy (both local and systemic). These complications may be managed by making changes in the dose or type of insulin used.

Choice of Pharmacologic Agent

Clearly, the choice of pharmacologic intervention for type II diabetes is a gray area. The choice between insulin and oral agents should be made with the particular patient in mind, taking into account the total clinical context of the patient's disease, acceptance of the various therapeutic modalities, level of diabetes education, and motivation. As a general guide, you may consider the opinion of the contributing editors and specialists in diabetes who reviewed the *Guide* before publication. They were given the chance to indicate their preferences in terms of pharmacologic therapy for several different hypothetical patients. The results of this informal survey are presented in Table 14.

Combination Therapy: Insulin Plus Oral Agent

When sulfonylurea drugs are effective as antidiabetic agents, they exert their effects, in large part, by increasing insulin action. Because of this, one might ask whether there is some indication for combining insulin and sulfonylurea therapy in the same patient. This may be an appropriate question if the patient has severe cellular resistance to insulin action.

Currently, the only candidate for combination therapy may be the patient in whom glycemic control cannot be achieved with diet and sulfonylurea therapy and in whom reasonable glycemic control cannot be achieved with two injections of mixed intermediate-acting and regular insulin each day. Although combination therapy has not been tested extensively, it appears that some patients of this type may respond to combination therapy with significant lowering of plasma glucose when an oral hypoglycemic agent is added to their only partially effective insulin treatment. Because this clinical problem is reasonably complicated, and because the efficacy of combination therapy still remains unproven, it is probably wise to refer the patient with refractory hyperglycemia to a specialist in diabetes.

Special Therapeutic Problems

Pregnancy and surgery in patients with diabetes mellitus are complicating situations that require extraordinary care to protect the patient against additional problems.

Pregnancy

Pregnancy can cause clinical difficulties for both the patient and her unborn baby. The infant of a diabetic mother has an increased risk of death, prematurity, and morbidity (congenital defects, macrosomia, hyperbilirubinemia, and respiratory distress syndrome). The diabetic mother faces an increased risk of ketoacidosis and hypoglycemia as

---

Table 14. Therapeutic Approach to Patients With Type II Diabetes Mellitus

This table presents results of a poll involving contributing editors and reviewing specialists in diabetes for the Guide.* However, it does not represent the opinion of all experts. Treatment must be INDIVIDUALIZED for all patients. In nearly all patient categories, there was disagreement, indicated by either/or. The weight of opinion is indicated as follows: blue capital letters, unanimous; blue and black capital letters, slight preference indicated in blue; blue capitals and black lowercase letters, preference indicated in capitals; black lowercase letters, no distinct preference.

FASTING PLASMA GLUCOSE (mg/dl)	AGE OF PATIENT (yr)			
	20	**40**	**60**	**80**
Obese Patient (Initial dietary treatment)				
115–139	DIET	DIET	DIET	diet or do nothing
140–199	ORAL AGENT or insulin	ORAL AGENT or insulin	ORAL AGENT	oral agent or diet
200+	INSULIN or oral agent	INSULIN or ORAL AGENT	ORAL AGENT or insulin	oral agent or insulin or diet
Nonobese Patient (Initial dietary treatment)				
115–139	INSULIN or oral agent	ORAL AGENT or insulin	ORAL AGENT	oral agent or diet
140–199	INSULIN	INSULIN or ORAL AGENT	ORAL AGENT or INSULIN	ORAL AGENT or INSULIN
200+	INSULIN	INSULIN or ORAL AGENT	INSULIN or oral agent	INSULIN or oral agent

*There was and is much disagreement among diabetes specialists concerning therapetic approaches expressed in this poll, including the authors and consultants to the *Guide.*

well as acceleration of microvascular complications involving the kidneys, eyes, and nervous system, particularly if hypertension is present.

In a patient with diabetes mellitus, pregnancy ideally should be planned so that conception occurs when the patient has normal fasting, preprandial, and postprandial plasma glucose levels. After conception, treatment should not only continue to achieve proper control of glycemia but also meet the nutritional requirements of the fetus. If the patient is being treated with a sulfonylurea agent, she should be switched to insulin during pregnancy.

Because the risks of pregnancy in association with diabetes mellitus are so great and involve both mother and fetus/newborn, and the treatment program (multiple injections of insulin or use of the insulin pump and euglycemic regulation) is so complex, the care of a pregnant diabetic woman should involve appropriate specialists. Consultation with personnel at a regionalized tertiary care program should be sought before conception, and referral of the patient should be seriously considered if the plasma glucose level exceeds 120 mg/dl at any time during pregnancy. Goals for glycemic control in diabetic women during pregnancy and normal glycosylated hemoglobin and plasma glucose levels are as follows:
■ fasting plasma glucose (60–90 mg/dl),
■ preprandial plasma glucose (<105 mg/dl), and
■ postprandial plasma glucose (<120 mg/dl).

Clearly, the physician in charge of a diabetic patient who contemplates pregnancy should inform the patient of the risks and possible need for referral. The physician who assumes responsibility for such a patient must be completely familiar with proper management of the patient and her fetus/newborn during pregnancy, just before and during delivery, and immediately after delivery.

The same vigorous attention to glycemic regulation and proper management of the patient and her fetus/newborn must be given to the individual who develops gestational diabetes during the second or third trimester.

Surgery

It is now possible for a patient with di-abetes mellitus to undergo surgical operations with little more than normal risk, unless the operation is done under emergency conditions that do not allow complete evaluation and preparation of the patient. What constitutes proper management of the diabetic surgical candidate should be of concern to the physician in charge of a patient with type II diabetes mellitus, because conditions requiring surgery often develop in older people in general and in diabetic patients in particular (e.g., occlusive vascular disease, gallbladder disease, cataract).

Unless the surgical condition is an emergency, the patient should be allowed sufficient time to achieve the best possible general health and control of hyperglycemia before admission to a hospital.

If possible, the patient should have a complete evaluation of metabolic state and thorough assessment of diabetic complications, including renal and heart disease, before surgery.

The objectives of management before, during, and after an operation are to prevent hypoglycemia, which can lead to coma, and to prevent excessive hyperglycemia and ketoacidosis, which can complicate postoperative care. To accomplish these ends, the anesthetic technique (regional or general) and the anesthetic agent should disrupt metabolic control as little as possible. Special attention should be given to maintaining proper fluid and electrolyte balance and blood glucose levels. In this regard, diabetic patients often need insulin therapy for control of hyperglycemia during the acute stress period of a major surgical procedure.

In the past few years, an increasing number of authorities have begun to advocate intravenous infusion of insulin instead of subcutaneous administration. In doing so, they note that intravenous administration circumvents problems of insulin delivery in the event of peripheral shutdown (hypotension, shock), which might occur during major surgery. Furthermore, intravenous administration makes it possible to carefully control the amount and speed of insulin delivery. With either administration technique, the operative team should understand the management objectives and work together to achieve them. In this critical effort, it is particularly important to involve an anesthesiologist who is trained in the management of diabetic patients.

To assume responsibility for the management of patients with type II diabetes during and after surgical procedures, the clinician must learn specific techniques involved in preparing the patient for surgery and for managing the patient during and after the operation. These techniques are described in textbooks on diabetes (see Bibliography).

The major principles governing the management of surgical candidates on the day of operation are presented in Table 15.

ASSESSMENT OF THE EFFICACY OF TREATMENT

Many diseases have a specific parameter that can be measured to determine the efficacy of therapy. This is not true in diabetes mellitus, because the metabolism of all body fuels (fat, carbohydrate, and protein) is deranged in this disease. In clinical practice, however, the therapeutic response to treatment of diabetes mellitus is monitored by determining effects on glucose metabolism. Specifically, the degree of blood glucose control is documented with a variety of direct and indirect techniques employed by the clinician and the patient.

In general, physicians assess blood glucose control with determinations of fasting, preprandial, and postprandial plasma glucose levels and with assays for glycosylated hemoglobin. Patients can determine the effects of therapy with self-monitoring of blood glucose as well as measurement of urine ketones, if necessary. Some patients also keep a daily diary in which they record food intake, meal plan, doses of insulin or oral hypoglycemic drugs, symptoms, and the results of self-administered urine and blood tests.

Monitoring of diabetes therapy may be as intense or as lax as the various forms of therapy. The frequency of patient visits, for instance, cannot be dictated. Most often, patients are seen fairly frequently after initiating treatment. In some cases, initial visits are used for the purpose of determining the degree of lability of blood glucose; in other cases, they are used to reinforce the necessity of following the therapeutic plan.

Table 15. Major Principles Governing Management of Diabetic Patients During Surgery in Hospitals and in Ambulatory Care Centers

■ The general management goals are to prevent hypoglycemia and ketoacidosis, to control hyperglycemia, to maintain normal electrolyte and fluid balance, and to resume oral feedings as soon as possible.

■ Ideally, plasma glucose level should be kept in the range of 115 to 140 mg/dl at all times. This kind of control requires constant vigilance to prevent hypoglycemia. Management is considered satisfactory when random plasma glucose levels during and after operation are between 150 and 250 mg/dl. Clearly, the clinician in charge must make judgments about target plasma glucose levels, taking into consideration skill and availability of the operative/postoperative team.

■ Plasma glucose levels should be determined frequently in perioperative period as a guide to therapy; urine glucose levels are unreliable. Usual recommendation is to obtain plasma glucose levels every 6 hours until patient resumes oral feeding, unless severe hyperglycemia necessitates more intense management.

■ Mild hyperglycemia is preferable to hypoglycemia. Thus, the smallest possible doses of insulin should be used to control hyperglycemia. Actual amount is determined by considering patient's plasma glucose levels before, during, and after operation, and, in the case of an insulin-taking patient, the usual insulin requirement.

■ Human or pork insulin should be used to cover patients who usually are not treated with insulin because they are less antigenic.

■ Operation should be scheduled for early morning, if possible.

The selection of self-monitoring methods depends on the individual patient. Self-monitoring always requires cooperation and intelligence on the part of the patient. Beyond that, the physician must consider the severity of the patient's illness as well as the patient's socioeconomic circumstances when recommending particular self-monitoring techniques.

Each of the assessment methods described below has advantages and disadvantages. Most often, a combination of methods is used to determine degree of metabolic control.

Office Methods

When a patient visits the office or clinic, the clinician can assess the degree of blood glucose control with a plasma glucose determination as well as with an assay for glycosylated hemoglobin. Both measurements are of value because the plasma glucose is an index of day-to-day control, whereas the glycosylated hemoglobin concentration reflects the level of glucose control for the preceding 2 months.

Plasma Glucose Determinations

Plasma glucose is an easily measured parameter that is a good reflection of metabolic control in a patient with relatively mild diabetes who visits the office every 1 or 2 months, provided that test results are interpreted correctly (i.e., taking into account the time of the last meal).

The major drawback to random plasma glucose determination, particularly in a patient with moderate to severe disease, is that it is difficult to know what a single blood glucose determination reflects. Even in patients with type II diabetes mellitus, blood glucose levels range widely during the day, so random determinations may simply represent peak values, trough values, or values in between. Furthermore, if the patient is visiting the office because of intercurrent illness, which frequently is the case, blood glucose levels will be of little value considering the fact that illness alters glucose tolerance. Also, some patients become more conscientious about following prescribed therapy just before office visits, in which case the plasma glucose level may be misleading.

Because plasma glucose levels never truly reflect the degree of chronic glucose control, they should be supplemented from time to time with an assay for glycosylated hemoglobin.

Glycosylated Hemoglobin Concentration

The glycosylated hemoglobin assay indicates the percentage of total hemoglobin to which glucose is attached. In some laboratories the measurement may be expressed as a percentage of hemoglobin A_1; in others it is expressed as a percentage of any one of the hemoglobin A_1 fractions (A_{1a}, A_{1b}, or A_{1c}, which is the largest). In some laboratories, for instance, the normal nondiabetic value for glycosylated hemoglobin may be 6.5 percent of total hemoglobin A_1, which is comparable to a mean plasma glucose level of 90 mg/dl.

Some specialists in diabetes consider the glycosylated hemoglobin level more important than an isolated plasma glucose level, because the latter is a single point in a fluctuating line and the former provides an index of the average. With the concept that glycosylation of other proteins may be the basis of the microangiopathy and the neuropathy of diabetes, the glycosylated hemoglobin concentration may even be an index of the predisposition to these complications.

If glycosylated hemoglobin is used as a means of assessing glucose control, it is important to know the laboratory norms and variations because these will influence interpretation of reported values. Commercial and hospital laboratories often use different techniques with various degrees of precision. It is also important to consider certain conditions that cause false elevations of glycosylated hemoglobin. These conditions include uremia, aspirin intake, the presence of fetal hemoglobin, and alcoholism. The conditions that cause falsely low levels of glycosylated hemoglobin include uremia, anemia, and variant hemoglobins, including HbS, C, and D, as well as active erythropoiesis, as occurs in pregnancy.

Given these precautions, an assay for glycosylated hemoglobin provides an index of the mean glucose levels to which tissues have been exposed for the previous several weeks and, as such, is an extremely valuable indicator of the level of chronic glucose control. The assay does not depend on patient cooperation and is not greatly affected by the day-to-day fluctuations in blood glucose levels.

A glycosylated hemoglobin concentration may be used to assess the effects of changes in therapy made 4 to 8 weeks earlier. It should not be used in the insulin-treated individual to determine the need for short-term changes in treatment. Blood glucose levels are still the means by which hour-to-hour and day-to-day changes in management are determined.

Home Methods

Between office visits, the patient can determine the degree of metabolic control by self-monitoring of glucose levels in blood, by testing the urine for ketones

Table 16. Products Available for Self-Monitoring of Blood Glucose

FINGER-STICKING SUPPLIES

Name and Manufacturer/ Distributor	Supplies and Features
Autoclix (Boehringer Mannheim)	Flat design; comes with 3 platforms to vary depth of penetration, 25 lancets
Auto-Lancet (Palco or Orange Medical Instruments)	Comes with 1 adult, 1 juvenile tip (guard), 2 lancets, case. Guard screws on
Autolet (Ames or Ulster Scientific)	Ulster: comes with 20 platforms (10 each of 2 different depths) Ames: comes with 10 platforms (regular depth), 10 lancets, plastic wallet
B-D Autolance (Becton Dickinson)	Flat design; one-piece construction; uses only Microfine lancets specially designed for this unit
Glucolet (Ames)	Comes with 10 Unilet lancets, regular puncture endcaps, super puncture endcaps, instruction insert
Monoject Lancet Device (Sherwood Medical)	Comes with bag of 5 endcaps or box with 10 endcaps; premeasured puncture depth
Penlet (LifeScan)	Clear guard; puncture depth controlled by amount of pressure applied by user
Monoject Lancets (Sherwood Medical)	
Easy Stik (Diabetes Supplies)	Can be used alone or in each of the above units except Autolance
TrendsLancets (Orange Medical Instruments)	
Glucosystem Lancets (Ames)	Can be used in either Autolet or Glucolet

TEST STRIPS FOR VISUAL READING

Name and Manufacturer	Instructions for Use
Chemstrip bG (Boehringer Mannheim)	Wipe after 1 minute, read; if >240, wait an additional minute, read
Glucostix (Ames)	Blot after 30 seconds, wait 90 seconds, read
TrendStrips (Orange Medical Instruments)	Wipe after 1 minute, read; if over 240, wait an additional minute, read
Visidex II* (Ames)	Blot after 30 seconds, wait 90 seconds, read

BLOOD GLUCOSE METERS

Name and Manufacturer	Test Strip Used	Range (mg/dl)
Accu-Chek II (Boehringer Mannheim)	Chemstrip bG	20–500
BetaScan Audio (Orange Medical Instruments)	TrendStrips	0–400
BetaScan B (Orange Medical Instruments)	TrendStrips	0–400
Diascan-S (Home Diagnostics)	Diascan	10–600
Diatron (Diatron Biomedical)	Diatron	11–432
Glucochek SC (EquiMed Medical Products)	Chemstrip bG	10–400
Glucochek SC Audio (EquiMed Medical Products)	Chemstrip bG	10–400
Glucometer II (Ames)	Glucostix	25–399
Glucometer II with memory (Ames)	Glucostix	25–399
Glucometer M (Ames)	Glucostix	25–399
Glucoscan 2000 (LifeScan)	Glucoscan test strips	25–450
Glucoscan 3000 (LifeScan)	Glucoscan test strips	25–450
Tracer (Boehringer Mannheim)	Tracer strips	40–400
TrendsMeter (Orange Medical Instruments)	TrendStrips	0–396

*For visual reading only, other strips listed above can be used with meter or read visually.

when necessary, and by keeping a daily record of therapy and test results.

Blood Glucose Monitoring
With the advent of self-monitoring of blood glucose, euglycemia has become a realistic goal for some patients with diabetes mellitus. Blood glucose monitoring is considerably more reliable than urine glucose tests for the detection of hyperglycemia and provides assurance against episodes of hypoglycemia.

Self-monitoring of blood glucose is particularly recommended for patients with marked insulin deficiency, such as those with labile blood glucose levels and those using split and mixed doses of insulin. Advocates of blood glucose self-monitoring also believe that patients with mild diabetes should employ this assessment method during periods of stress, such as those caused by infection or trauma, as well as to periodically reinforce their commitment to the prescribed therapeutic plan.

All of the available products (Table 16) include the use of a reagent strip that develops a color reaction to the glucose in the patient's blood. The use of an automated lance for finger stick is recommended. After coloration occurs, the strip can be compared to a color chart by the patient or it can be read by a reflectance meter that provides a numerical value for blood glucose.

Self-tested blood glucose results can tell patients if their blood glucose is low, normal, or high. Self-monitoring of blood glucose truly involves patients in the treatment of their disease. With proper instructions, the patient can be taught to make adjustments in therapy based on test results.

Some advocates of blood glucose self-monitoring for patients with type II diabetes suggest that the patient should determine blood glucose levels four times a day initially (before each meal and at bedtime). After a stable pattern is established, they suggest that the patient measure the prebreakfast level three to seven times a week and also obtain a preprandial profile of four measurements between one and three times a month. In addition, because patients with type II diabetes often have lengthy postprandial elevations of glucose and should postpone the next meal until after the blood glucose returns to normal, self-monitoring is useful for determining the appropriate interval between meals. Patients with self-monitoring equipment should increase frequency of determinations during illness and other conditions of stress.

Urine Glucose Determinations
The determination of urine glucose has, for the most part, been superceded by self-measurements of blood glucose. Urinary glucose measurements are indirect and are not precise, and they should be reserved for patients who cannot or will not perform self-monitoring of blood glucose.

Urine Ketone Determinations
Urine ketone determinations are mandatory when the patient has significant hyperglycemia or is symptomatic, because it is the only indication of impending ketoacidosis.

Patient Record
The patient should be encouraged to keep a daily record of food intake, doses of insulin or oral hypoglycemic drug, symptoms (including the time and circumstances), and the results of all blood testing. The main effect of this record is positive reinforcement of the importance of therapy. Indeed, this type of record is very important for the overweight individual, because the requirement to document food eaten during the day often helps patients to modify their eating habits and to initiate weight reduction. The daily diary is particularly important if the patient has labile diabetes or is taking insulin.

The patient record is helpful to the physician because it indicates the patient's degree of interest in control and provides information necessary for development of effective therapeutic plans.

BIBLIOGRAPHY

Therapeutic Objectives and Plan

DeFronzo RA, Ferrannini E, Koivisto V: New concepts in the pathogenesis and treatment of noninsulin dependent diabetes mellitus. *Am J Med* 74:52–81, 1983

Gordon T, Castelli WP, Hjortland MC, et al: Diabetes, blood lipids and the role of obesity in CHD risk for women: the Framingham study. *Ann Intern Med* 87:393–97, 1977

Dietary Modification

American Diabetes Association: Nutritional recommendations and principles for individuals with diabetes mellitus, 1986. *Diabetes Care* 10:126–32, 1987

Anderson JW, Ward K: Long-term effects of high carbohydrate, high fiber diets on glucose and lipid metabolism: preliminary report on patients with diabetes. *Diabetes Care* 1:77–82, 1978

Arky RA: Nutritional management of the diabetic. In *Diabetes Mellitus: Theory and Practice*. 3rd ed. Ellenberg M, Rifken H, Eds. New Hyde Park, NY, Medical Examination Publishing, 1983, chapt. 26

Crapo PA: A survey of sweeteners (Abstract). *Clinical Diabetes* 1:21, 1983

Crapo PA: Dietary modification in the management of diabetes. In *Handbook of Diabetes Mellitus, Clinical and Experimental Aspects*. Vol. V. Brownlee M, Ed. New York, Garland STPM, 1981

Davidson JK: A new look at diet therapy. *Diabetes Forecast* May/June:14–19, 1976

Food and Nutrition Board, National Research Council: *Recommended Dietary Allowances*. 9th ed. Washington, DC, National Academy of Sciences, 1980

Hadden DR: Food and diabetes: the dietary treatment of insulin-dependent and non-insulin-dependent diabetes. *Clin Endocrinol Metab* 11:503–23, 1982

West KM: Diet therapy of diabetes: an analysis of failure. *Ann Intern Med* 79:425–34, 1973

Wing RR: Improving dietary adherence in patients with diabetes. In *Contemporary Issues in Nutrition: Nutrition and Diabetes*. Jovanovic L, Petersen CM, Eds. New York, Liss, 1985

Appropriate Physical Activity

Björntorp P, Berchtold P, Grimby G, et al: Effects of physical training on glucose tolerance, plasma insulin and lipids and on body composition in men after myocardial infarction. *Acta Med Scand* 192:439–43, 1972

Björntorp P, de Jounge K, Sjöström L, et al: Physical training in human obesity. II. Effects of plasma insulin in glucose intolerant subjects without marked hyperinsulinemia. *Scand J Clin Lab Invest* 32:42–45, 1973

Björntorp P, de Jounge K, Sjöström L, et al: The effect of physical training on insulin production in obesity. *Metabolism* 19:631–37, 1970

Björntorp P, Fahler M, Grimby G, et al: Carbohydrate and lipid metabolism in middle aged physically well-trained men. *Metabolism* 21:1037–42, 1972

Gustafson A: Effect of training on blood lipids. In *Coronary Heart Disease and Physical Fitness*. Larson OA, Malmborg RO, Eds. Copenhagen, Munksgaard, 1971, p. 125–29

Holloszy JO, Skinner JS, Toro G, et al: Effects of a six month program of endurance exercise on the serum lipids of middle-aged men. *Am J Cardiol* 14:753–60, 1964

Horton ES: Diet, muscle metabolism, and capacity for exercise in obesity. In *Recent Advances in Obesity Research II. Proceedings of the Second International Congress on Obesity*. Bray G, Ed. London, Newman, 1978, chapt. 33

Horton ES: The role of exercise in the treatment of hypertension in obesity. *Int J Obes* 5 (Suppl. 1):165–71, 1981

Huttunen JK, Lansimies E, Voutilainen E, et al: Effect of moderate physical exercise on serum high density lipoproteins. *Circulation* 60:1220–29, 1979

Koivisto VA, Felig P: Exercise in diabetes: clinical implications. In *Diabetes Mellitus*. Vol. V. Rifkin H, Raskin P, Eds. Bowie, MD, Brady, 1981, chapt. 16

Lipman RL, Raskin P, Love T, et al: Glucose intolerance during decreased physical activity in man. *Diabetes* 21:101–107, 1972

Pyörälä K: Relationship of glucose tolerance and plasma insulin to the incidence of coronary heart disease: results from two population studies in Finland. *Diabetes Care* 2:131–41, 1979

Richter EA, Ruderman NB, Schneider SH: Diabetes and exercise. *Am J Med* 70:201–209, 1981

Ruderman NB, Ganda OP, Johansen K: The effect of physical training on glucose tolerance and plasma lipids in maturity-onset diabetes. *Diabetes* 28 (Suppl. 1):89–92, 1979

Saltin B, Lindgärde F, Houston M, Hörlin R, Nygaard E, Gad P: Physical training and glucose tolerance in middle-aged men with chemical diabetes. *Diabetes* 28 (Suppl. 1):30–32, 1979

Siegel W, Blomqvist G, Mitchell JH: Effects of a quantitative physical training program on middle-aged sedentary men. *Circulation* 41:19–29, 1970

Vranic M, Kemmer FW, Berchtold P, et al: Hormonal interaction in control of metabolism during exercise in physiology and diabetes. In *Diabetes Mellitus: Theory and Practice*. 3rd ed. Ellenberg M, Rifkin H, Eds. New Hyde Park, NY, Medical Examination Publishing, 1983, chapt. 27

Welborn TA, Wearne K: Coronary heart disease incidence and cardiovascular mortality in Busselton with reference to glucose and insulin concentrations. *Diabetes Care* 2:154–60, 1979

Zinman B: Exercise in diabetes treatment. *Clin Diabetes* 1:18–21, 1983

Pharmacologic Intervention

Clinical Use of Oral Hypoglycemic Agents

Groop L, Wahlin-Boll E, Groop PH, et al: Pharmacokinetics and metabolic effects of glibenclamide and glipizide in type 2 diabetics. *Eur J Clin Pharmacol* 28:697–704, 1985

Lebovitz HE: Oral hypoglycemic agents. In *The Diabetes Annual/1*. Alberti KGMM, Krall LP, Eds. Amsterdam, Elsevier, 1985, p. 93–110

Lebovitz HE: Oral hypoglycemic agents. In *The Diabetes Annual/3*. Alberti KGMM, Krall LP, Eds. Amsterdam, Elsevier, 1987, p. 72–93

Lebovitz HE, Feinglos MN: The oral hypoglycemic agents. In *Diabetes Mellitus: Theory and Practice*. 3rd ed. Ellenberg M, Rifkin H, Eds. New Hyde Park, NY, Medical Examination Publishing, 1983, chapt. 28

Melander A: Clinical pharmacology of sulfonylureas. *Metabolism* 36 (Suppl. 1):12–16, 1987

Whitehouse FW, Kahkonen DM: Oral hypoglycemic agents. In *Diabetes Mellitus*. Vol. V. Rifkin H, Raskin P, Eds. Bowie, MD, Brady, 1981, chapt. 15

Clinical Use of Insulin

Furth FG, Bell PM, Rizza RA: Effects of tolazamide and exogenous insulin on insulin action in patients with non-insulin-dependent diabetes mellitus. *N Engl J Med* 314:1280–86, 1986

Galloway JA, de Shazo RD: The clinical use of insulin and the complications of insulin therapy. In *Diabetes Mellitus: Theory and Practice*. 3rd ed. Ellenberg M, Rifkin H, Eds. New Hyde Park, NY, Medical Examination Publishing, 1983

Karam JH: Insulins 1983: overview and outlook (Abstract). *Clin Diabetes* 1:10, 1983

Multicenter Study: U.K. Prospective diabetes study. II. Reduction in HbA$_{1c}$ with basal insulin supplement, sulfonylurea, or biquanide therapy in maturity-onset diabetes. *Diabetes* 34:793–98, 1985

Multi-Centre Study: UK prospective study of therapies of maturity-onset diabetes. I. Effect of diet, sulphonylurea, insulin or biguanide therapy on fasting plasma glucose and body weight over one year. *Diabetologia* 24:404–11, 1983

Scarlett JA, Gray RS, Griffin J, et al: Insulin treatment reserves the insulin resistance of type II diabetes mellitus. *Diabetes Care* 5:353–63, 1983

Stout RW: Is insulin atherogenic: *Mt Sinai J Med* 49:223–26, 1982

University Group Diabetes Program: Effects of hypoglycemic agents on vascular complications in patients with adult-onset diabetes. VIII. Evaluation of insulin therapy: final report. *Diabetes* 31 (Suppl. 5):1–26, 1982

Special Therapeutic Problems

Pregnancy

National Diabetes Advisory Board: *The Prevention and Treatment of Five Complications of Diabetes: A Guide for Primary Care Practitioners.* Washington, DC, U.S. Department of Health and Human Services, 1983. NIH publ. no. 82-8392

Proceedings of the Second International Workshop-Conference on Gestational Diabetes Mellitus: *Diabetes* 34: Suppl. 2, 1985

Surgery

Shuman CR: Surgery and diabetes. In *Diabetes Mellitus: Theory and Practice.* 3rd ed. Ellenberg M, Rifkin H, Eds. New Hyde Park, NY, Medical Examination Publishing, 1983, chapt. 33

Sussman KE, Kolterman OG: Surgery in the patient with diabetes. In *Diabetes Mellitus.* Vol. V. Rifkin H, Raskin P, Eds. Bowie, MD, Brady, 1981, chapt. 26

Assessment of the Efficacy of Treatment

Concensus statement on self-monitoring of blood glucose. *Diabetes Care* 10:95–99, 1987

Gabbay KH, Flückiger R: Clinical significance of glycosylated hemoglobin. In *Diabetes Mellitus.* Vol. V. Rifkin H, Raskin P, Eds. Bowie, MD, Brady, 1981, chapt. 28

Nathan DM: Glycosylated hemoglobin: what it is and how to use it. *Clin Diabetes* 1:1–7, 1983

Self-monitoring methods for blood glucose. *Med Lett Drugs Ther* 25:42–44, 1983

Skyler JS: Patient self-monitoring of blood glucose. *Clin Diabetes* 1:12–17, 1983

Techniques for Helping the Patient Cope With Diagnosis and Treatment

Highlights

Some patients react to diabetes with denial, anger, hostility, or depression before acceptance of the challenges that diabetes implies. By acknowledging and understanding these patient reactions, the physician provides the patient with emotional support, one of the key ingredients for patient compliance.

Along with understanding the many concerns of the diabetic patient (pages 57–63), the physician should be aware of the following:

■ the determinants of compliance (Table 17, page 62),

■ the common reasons for failure of patients to adhere to recommended therapeutic plans (Table 18, page 62), and

■ specific techniques that may be used to enhance compliance (Table 19, page 63).

The clinician can enhance patient compliance by

■ determining the patient's health-care beliefs and correcting misconceptions as necessary (see Health-Care Beliefs Related to Diabetes, page 58),

■ providing the patient with adequate education and technical skills,

■ guiding the patient in making changes in behavior,

■ tailoring the therapeutic regimen to the patient's life-style,

■ working with the patient to set mutual goals,

■ encouraging the patient's efforts,

■ praising the patient's success, and

■ enlisting help from other health-care professionals and patient support groups.

Techniques for Helping the Patient Cope With Diagnosis and Treatment

INTRODUCTION

Until recently, little emphasis was placed on the importance of treating patients with type II diabetes. In the past, these patients, who account for about 90 percent of all diabetic people in the United States, were not given adequate attention because the disease usually does not cause significant symptoms, and many physicians found it frustrating to deal with middle-aged to elderly, generally obese, seemingly disinterested patients.

Today, attitudes are different. Because of the increasing emphasis on wellness through proper diet and exercise in general, physicians are giving these therapeutic tools more attention. Circuitously, the patient with type II diabetes is benefiting from the enlightenment of physicians. Furthermore, the receptiveness of at least some patients to recommendations for life-style change is enabling the necessary partnership for management to develop more easily.

Because type II diabetes generally is diagnosed at a time in the patient's life when behavior patterns have been established, the requirements to learn new eating habits and to incorporate exercise into the daily schedule are very difficult. Added to that is a need for self-monitoring of blood glucose, collecting and testing of urine, record keeping, regular visits to the physician, and attendance at educational programs, making the difficulty an intrusion. In addition, the patients have concerns about complications, a shortened life, the attitudes of family and friends, and, for some, the effect on employment and insurance. It is no wonder, therefore, that the individual with type II diabetes mellitus experiences a range of emotions that need to be appreciated and dealt with by the physician.

The following discussion is intended to provide the physician with an understanding of patients with type II diabetes. With this understanding, the clinician should be better prepared to help the patient and family cope with the diagnosis and treatment. This discussion also presents the issues involved in patient compliance with recommended treatment plans, i.e., the determinants of compliance, the common reasons for noncompliance, and techniques for enhancing compliance.

PATIENT RESPONSES TO DIAGNOSIS AND TREATMENT

The physician should anticipate any one of a number of different reactions from the patient with diabetes. Before accepting the numerous challenges that the diagnosis of diabetes mellitus implies, it is not unusual for some patients to react with denial, anger, hostility, or depression. The physician who is sensitive to these reactions and who acknowledges an understanding of them is providing a supportive environment for the patient, which is one key factor encouraging patient compliance.

FACTORS THAT INFLUENCE THE PATIENT'S EMOTIONAL RESPONSE TO DIABETES

A patient's emotional responses to diabetes are deeply intertwined with a number of factors, including age at the time of diagnosis, basic personality, self-image, health-care beliefs, and social and economic environment.

Age at Time of Diagnosis

The implications of diabetes are different for elderly and middle-aged individuals. An elderly patient, who may be isolated socially and who may already be experiencing progressive physical impairments, will often consider the suggestion of an alteration in life-style to be threatening to security. A middle-

Health-Care Beliefs Related to Diabetes

The patient's emotional response to diagnosis and treatment of diabetes mellitus and willingness to follow prescribed therapy depend in large measure on health-care beliefs.

To enhance success with prescribed therapy, the clinician should determine the patient's health-care beliefs and try to correct misconceptions before outlining the therapeutic plan.

It is important to determine the patient's attitudes about the following:

Susceptibility to the disease

Possible response (denial): "I hear what you are saying, but no one in my family has diabetes, and I feel great. The laboratory probably made a mistake."

Consequences of the disease

Possible response (indifference): "I hear what you are saying, but so what? My dad has diabetes, and he's just fine. I feel great."

Value of treatment

Possible response (futility): "I believe you, but nothing can be done about the disease. I have a relative with diabetes who tried hard and did just what the doctor told him to do. He had a heart attack anyway."

Risk vs. benefits of treatment

Possible response (defeat): "I believe that I have the disease, but what you are telling me to do will ruin my life. Isn't there another way?"

Basic Personality, Self-Image, and Health-Care Beliefs

There is no "diabetic personality." Diabetes happens to people, and, although it introduces a new set of problems, the patient's usual pattern of response to challenge can be expected to prevail. There may be willingness to accept personal responsibility or a need to shift responsibility entirely to someone else, in this case, the health-care provider.

Individual patient reaction also depends on the patient's self-image and perception of the importance of health. The patient's responses are further influenced by beliefs about the cause and treatment of disease.

Social and Economic Environment

The patient who is unmarried and without close family may find the diagnosis frightening because it reinforces the feeling of aloneness. On the other hand, the patient who has the support of family and friends receives positive reinforcement and finds that the new requirements for living can be more easily integrated into daily schedules.

Economic factors may influence the patient's emotional response to diabetes as well because of the inability to afford proper food, prescribed medication, and medical care.

SPECIFIC THERAPEUTIC ISSUES OF SIGNIFICANCE TO THE PATIENT

There are a number of specific therapeutic issues that have special significance to the patient with type II diabetes mellitus. Some of the more important issues are the need to lose weight, to increase physical activity, to monitor blood and urine glucose, and to make frequent visits to the physician and other health-care professionals. Patients may also fear complications of diabetes.

In addition, the physician who empathizes with the patient should experience less anger and frustration at patient noncompliance and be able to tolerantly and tirelessly encourage the patient to work toward desired therapeutic goals. With this kind of relationship between physician and patient, the

aged patient also may find this health problem threatening but for different reasons. In the younger individual, the diagnosis calls attention to mortality and presents a new and totally unexpected obstacle in life. Instead of being able to coast along in well-established routines, the patient with diabetes has to take time off from work to visit the physician and make other major changes in lifestyle. If the person is going through a midlife crisis such as career change or divorce, the diagnosis is an extra burden.

burden of failure to achieve therapeutic goals is removed from the physician and reduced in the patient, and the chances for eventual compliance are increased.

Weight Reduction

Because most individuals with type II diabetes are obese, and because there is no doubt that weight reduction is extremely important in reducing blood glucose levels, it is critical that physicians be prepared to understand the problems faced by obese patients.

In the treatment of type II diabetes, the problem of losing weight is significant. Much has been written about the psychodynamics of obesity, and research in recent years offers helpful information about why it may be more difficult metabolically for people with type II diabetes to lose weight. Whatever the reason, successful weight reduction is not an easy accomplishment for these patients.

A frequent scenario is immediate weight loss attributable to patient enthusiasm and physician encouragement, which is quickly followed by a plateau or slight regain of weight, boredom, frustration, and failure. During this process, one of the most difficult experiences for the patient is to face the physician when expected results have not been achieved. The weight scales and blood glucose levels document failure that the patient cannot escape.

The physician who understands what the patient is feeling can become a motivator and turn the patient's feelings of frustration, anger, and futility into sustained action and ultimate behavioral changes that lead to long-term success.

When weight reduction is a goal, the physician should never be judgmental or accusatory. The physician should always provide positive reinforcement and assurance that a little success is better than none at all and that persistence will bring success.

Because even slight weight loss is often followed by significant reductions in blood glucose, it is not necessary to discourage a patient by setting unreachable short-term goals. The physician should not try too much too soon and should verbalize that it is hard to lose weight and that it *is* a deprivation when others can eat more without having to worry about a blood glucose level.

The obstacles to successful weight reduction are many. Eating is a pleasurable experience. Food is appealing. Social situations revolve around food. The physician should explain to the patient that restaurant eating and social dining are possible but require thought about the selection of foods. The patient should be told that most restaurants are able to prepare food with attention to special needs. In a situation where the type or amount of food is a problem, the patient should be prepared to state that he/she is on a diet or has diabetes and must be careful about the food he/she eats. When necessary, the patient should be prepared to accept a problem situation by eating a small amount of "forbidden" food without guilt with the attitude that "tomorrow is another day."

It is important to individually treat each patient's weight problem. Some patients need absolute rules, whereas others prefer flexibility. Because there is no printed diet that fits every patient, it is important for the physician to incorporate a dietitian into the educational process and to know what the patient learns so that the dietary approach is coordinated.

Many clinicians encourage their patients to join support groups such as Overeaters Anonymous and to use special programs such as Weight Watchers and TOPS.

Above all, the clinician should express pleasure with patient success and be encouraging when progress is slow. It is the physician's responsibility to motivate patients when they become discouraged and apathetic and to help them establish new behavior patterns by making them feel good about their accomplishments.

Increased Physical Activity

Although diet and exercise are the cornerstones in the treatment plan for type II diabetes, there is tremendous patient resistance to both. Because most patients really do want to lose weight, those with diabetes are more willing to try dietary modifications than they are to engage in physical activity.

The excuses given by the patient are consistent. "I don't have time." "I get enough exercise running around in my work all day." "I'm too tired to exercise when I get home." "It's been too hot." "It's been too cold." "I just read that people drop dead from jogging."

Seldom do physicians hear the truth. Patients resent the discipline and regimentation that daily exercise implies; they are embarrassed because they are overweight, sometimes clumsy, and appear strange in athletic attire. Patients fear that they will fail to succeed in the programs prescribed.

As in diet therapy for weight reduction, the physician must be a motivator and stress the importance of incorporating exercise into the daily routine. If the physician does not take the need for exercise seriously, it is unlikely that the patient will.

Exercise should be considered a prescription, and the patient must be a participant in determining the dosage of exercise to be prescribed. When the clinician and patient establish a mutually agreed on therapeutic regimen, the patient is more likely to participate in the plan.

The clinician should keep in mind that even small amounts of exercise are acceptable and that motivating the patient to do something is better than nothing at all. The patient who starts with an activity that is possible will experience accomplishment, which often will be the catalyst for continued and increased physical activity.

Self-Monitoring of Urine and Blood Sugars

For years, urine testing and record keeping have been used by physicians to measure control of diabetes. The offensiveness and inconvenience of testing urine are continuing complaints. When urine testing was the principle method of monitoring, a patient's moods and attitudes often depended on the finding of a positive or negative urine glucose. Control was either "good" or "bad." Accusations of noncompliance were sometimes made on the basis of finding too much glucose in the urine.

Now, self-monitoring of blood glucose has entered the picture and is considered by many specialists in diabetes as one of the most important advances in clinical management. Self-monitoring is a mixed blessing, however. There is no question that knowledge of blood glucose level at any particular moment helps the patient to distinguish between uncertain sensations and to correctly attribute symptoms to hyperglycemia or to hypoglycemia. The old attitude "I can tell how my control is by the way I feel" has been disproved more than it has been supported by self-monitoring of blood glucose.

Nevertheless, some patients find the physical discomfort from sticking the finger for a drop of blood, the requirement for repetitive testing to obtain meaningful results, and the inconvenience associated with performing this test as disagreeable as urine testing.

Patients soon learn that documentation of blood glucose levels leaves no doubt about the current state of regulation as well as about the ongoing degree of control. The results of testing cause depression in many patients. In others, a documented failure leads to recognition of indiscretion and to guilt. Some patients experience feelings of futility with blood testing, because diligent efforts have not been rewarded with "good numbers."

Self-monitoring of blood glucose does document fact. When it is properly performed, it leaves no doubt about the level of control. Patients must be taught to understand that this monitoring method is a tool to help them make judgments about their own treatment. With the attitude that the technique puts them in charge of their program, patients should feel more positive about this aspect of treatment.

The physician should assist the patient in assessing the self-monitoring results and implementing appropriate changes. Judgments regarding good or bad results are self-defeating and play no constructive role in diabetes care.

Frequent Visits to the Physician and Other Health-Care Professionals

Diabetes requires regular visits to the physician and other health-care professionals. If the health-care providers' attitudes are positive, the experience for the patient will be useful and satisfying even if results of metabolic assessment are less than desired.

If health-care professionals convey the feeling that the needs and concerns of the patient are too time consuming or that therapeutic efforts are unlikely to be effective, the patient will consider these visits intrusions or negative experiences.

Complications of Diabetes

Individuals with diabetes fear the development of complications. If they do not know about them before they are diagnosed, it does not take long before they read or hear about blindness, amputations, kidney failure, and neuropathy. The patient's fear may be active, or it may be quiescent and controlled. Fear is always there, ready to surface when some alteration in status occurs.

A change in visual acuity resulting from erratic control is interpreted by the patient as impending blindness. A pain in the foot activates the fear of gangrene and amputation. A backache means kidney failure. An alteration in sexual performance signifies impotence.

The physician should anticipate these concerns and be willing to discuss the facts about complications with the patient and family so they feel comfortable in asking for help. Some physicians are reluctant to discuss prognosis or the possibility of developing complications because they do not want to upset the patient or family. The patient may be reluctant to talk about fears, and the family may even recognize developing complications but also hold back in expressing fear.

An honest presentation of the problems associated with diabetes and discussion of the current attitude that good control may delay the onset or prevent or improve complications are both reassuring and motivating to the patient and family. Telling the patient and family about new ways of treating complications also helps to allay their anxiety and fear.

Behavior Modification Strategies Applied to Weight Reduction

Behavior modification techniques applied to weight reduction may include some or all of the following.

Identify the stimuli that lead to eating, and encourage patient to eliminate those stimuli.

Traditional Measures
Have the patient

- remove food from sight;
- keep candy and cookies out of the house; and
- place low-calorie bulk vegetables in the front of refrigerator or in strategic places.

Other Measures
Tell the patient to

- avoid eating while watching TV, reading, or listening to the radio;
- eat in one place (no matter what is eaten);
- prepare a full table setting when eating any food (it slows the act of eating);
- use smaller plates;
- count each mouthful;
- place utensils on plate after every third mouthful; and
- have a 2-minute interruption before end of meal.

Use a point system for adherence, and encourage the patient to reward himself/herself (with money, gifts, vacation) after successfully accumulating a predetermined number of points.

Encourage the patient to take responsibility for his/her behavior and to become involved in self-monitoring. Ask the patient to keep a written record of the type, quantity, and caloric value of food eaten. This calls attention to eating habits.

Reinforce patient record keeping. Use graphs to show weight loss or gain. Alternatively, graph patient behaviors that lead to weight loss, e.g., number of places in which the patient eats or frequency of eating.

ISSUES IN PATIENT COMPLIANCE

Understanding the issues and concerns of the patient with diabetes and then conveying this understanding to the patient is the first step toward patient compliance. Understanding is not enough, however. To ensure good patient compliance, the physician should also know the determinants of compliance, the common reasons for failure, and some

Table 17. Determinants of Compliance

Factors that have been shown to be predictors of compliance include

- **Complexity of regimen**
  The greater the complexity, the less likely is compliance.
  Solution: simplify when possible.

- **Need to change behavior**
  The greater the need to change life-style, the less likely is compliance.
  Solution: Tailor therapeutic plan to patient's life-style as much as possible. Show patient how to incorporate favorite foods into meal plan, for instance.

- **Duration of treatment**
  The longer the treatment lasts, the less likely is compliance.

- **Clinician's communication skills**
  Physicians who communicate well are more likely to have patients who follow prescribed regimens. To be successful, patients must know what to do.

- **Quality of support system**
  Patients who have good support from family and health-care professionals are more likely to succeed than patients who are without social and medical support.

Table 18. Common Reasons for Failure of Patients to Comply With Treatment Plans

- **Lack of education about the disease and its treatment.** Patients who do not know what to do cannot comply with prescribed therapy.

- **Faulty health-care beliefs.** Patients will not comply with recommended therapeutic intervention unless convinced of its value.

- **Lack of necessary skills.** Patients who know *what* to do but not *how* to do it cannot comply with therapeutic plan.

- **Lack of adequate support from family, friends, and health-care professionals.** Patients who are "on their own" to accomplish therapeutic plans are unlikely to be successful.

specific techniques for enhancing compliance.

Determinants of Compliance

The determinants of compliance are presented in Table 17. Notice that the following factors are *not* considered predictive of compliance: level of education, intelligence, income, race, and sex. Instead, compliance is influenced by the complexity of the regimen, the need to change behavior, the duration of treatment, the communication skills of the clinician, and the quality of the support system for the patient.

Common Reasons for Noncompliance

In addition to the predictors of compliance, it is useful to know the common reasons for patient noncompliance (Table 18). The reasons generally include one or more of the following:
- the patient did not know what was expected of him/her;
- the patient knew what was expected but did not believe it was worth the effort;
- the patient knew what was expected but did not have the skills to perform required tasks; and
- the patient knew what was expected but did not have adequate support from family, friends, or health-care professionals.

Techniques for Enhancing Compliance

When one considers the determinants of compliance, it is easy to understand why diabetes is problematic. Of the five determinants of compliance, two—the need to change behavior and duration of treatment—are difficult to modify. Clinicians can, however, improve their own communication skills, simplify the regimen when possible, and improve the quality of the support system for the patient.

Specific techniques for enhancing compliance are outlined in Table 19. Most important, the clinician should begin the process by determining the patient's health-care beliefs. It is naive to assume that the patient is an "empty vessel." The clinician who asks appropriate questions knows where to begin correcting misconceptions (see Health-

Care Beliefs Related to Diabetes, page 58). After correcting health-care beliefs, the clinician should make certain the patient has all the information and skills necessary to follow prescribed plans. This step usually involves several other health-care professionals, including a diabetes educator, nutritionist, or dietitian.

The third technique for enhancing patient compliance is guidance in behavior modification. Again, the clinician may need help from outside professionals. An example of behavior modification technique as applied to weight reduction is provided on page 61.

The fourth technique for enhancing compliance involves the provision of a proper support system for the patient. The clinician should try to make the therapeutic plan as compatible with the patient's life-style as possible. For example, the dietary plan should allow for ethnic tastes. The clinician and patient should work together to set mutual goals. Some physicians advocate "contracting" and say that a written contract is better than an oral agreement. Finally, the clinician should always en-

courage the patient's efforts and should praise success. Given that the therapeutic regimen for diabetes can be overwhelmingly complex, the physician may start by focusing on one aspect of the regimen and then adding to the regimen as the patient adjusts.

Table 19. Techniques for Enhancing Patient Compliance

Physicians can assist patients in the following ways:

- determine patient's health-care beliefs and correct misconceptions as necessary (see Health-Care Beliefs Related to Diabetes, page 58);
- provide patient with adequate education and technical skills; and
- guide patient in making changes in behavior.

Provide a supportive environment in the following ways:

- tailor therapeutic regimen to patient's life-style;
- work with patient to set mutual goals, and consider a written contract; and
- encourage patient's efforts and praise success.

BIBLIOGRAPHY

Citron WS, Kleiman GA, Skyler JS: Emotions: a critical factor in diabetic control. In *Diabetes Mellitus: Diagnosis and Treatment.* Davidson MB, Ed. New York, Wiley, 1981, chapt. 9

Cohen SJ: Improving patients' compliance with therapeutic regimens. *J Indiana State Med Assoc* 76:26–29, 1983

Hamburg BA, Lipsett LF, Inoff GE, Drash AL, Eds. *Behavioral and Psychosocial Issues in Diabetes. Proceedings of the National Conference.* Washington, DC, U.S. Department of Health and Human Services. 1979, p. 229–32, 282–86 (NIH publ. no. 80-1993)

Jacobson AM, Hauser ST: Behavioral and psychological aspects of diabetes. In *Diabetes Mellitus: Theory and Practice.* 3rd ed. Ellenberg M, Rifkin H, Eds. New Hyde Park, NY, Medical Examination Publishing, 1983, p. 1038–39

Detection and Treatment of Complications of Type II Diabetes Mellitus

Highlights

Patients with diabetes are susceptible to numerous complications, both chronic and acute, as well as many adverse drug reactions.

The major risk factors for the macro- and microvascular complications of diabetes are
- hypertension
- hyperlipidemia
- hyperglycemia
- lack of exercise
- smoking

Most of the above risk factors are more prevalent in the type II diabetic population and act synergistically to promote vascular disease.

MAJOR CHRONIC COMPLICATIONS

Diabetic patients are twice as prone as nondiabetic individuals to die from coronary artery disease, and the average annual incidence of cardiovascular sequelae is increased at least twofold in patients with diabetes.

It is important to lower plasma lipid and glucose levels and to control hypertension, the latter being particularly important in terms of its benefits for reducing risks of microvascular (retinopathy and nephropathy) and macrovascular disease.

Diet and exercise programs should be utilized to help the patient achieve ideal weight. Cigarette smoking should cease.

Diabetic retinopathy does not cause visual symptoms until a fairly advanced stage has been reached, usually either macular edema or proliferative retinopathy.

The changes involved in diabetic retinopathy may be subtle and suggest that all patients with type II diabetes should have a complete evaluation by a practitioner skilled in the examination of the retina, including visual history, visual acuity examination, and careful ophthalmoscopic examination with dilated pupils at least once yearly.

A discussion of the clinical presentation of background and proliferative diabetic retinopathies is presented on pages 69–71.

The indications for referral to an ophthalmologist are summarized in Table 21, page 71.

Management of diabetic retinopathy is more satisfactory when intervention is undertaken before visual symptoms develop.

Hypertension is associated with increased incidence of diabetic retinopathy as well as an increased rate of progression of diabetic retinopathy and, therefore, must be treated. Potential complications with antihypertensive medications should be kept in mind (Table 22, page 72).

The ophthalmologic treatment of diabetic retinopathy depends on the stage of disease (page 70).

The incidence of diabetic renal disease is at least 5 to 10 percent 20 years after diagnosis in patients whose diabetes was diagnosed after age 30 (presumably type II).

To monitor the onset of renal disease, a urinalysis (including microscopic analysis), creatinine, and/or blood urea nitrogen should be done in all new patients. They should be repeated yearly in all patients.

Proteinuria usually is the first indication of renal disease.

To delay the onset and acceleration of renal disease, hypertension must be detected and treated.

Consultation with a specialist is suggested if persistent proteinurea, and elevation in serum creatinine or blood urea nitrogen, or hypertension unresponsive to treatment is seen.

More than 50 percent of the non-traumatic amputations in the United States occur in individuals with diabetes, and it has been estimated that more than half of these could have been prevented with proper care.

Early foot lesions often go undetected because they usually are painless.

The prevention of foot problems requires proper foot care by the patient as well as early detection and prompt treatment of lesions by the physician.

More serious foot problems are best handled in consultation with specialists in diabetic foot care.

The patient with proper instruction should assume major responsibility for prevention of foot problems. Minor noninfected wounds can be treated with nonirritating antiseptic solution, daily dressing changes, and foot rest.

The peripheral neuropathies include the symmetrical bilateral neuropathies of the upper and lower extremities, various specific mononeuropathies, neuropathic ulcer, and diabetic amyotrophy. Suggested approaches to management of these problems are presented on pages 73 to 75.

The autonomic neuropathies include gastroparesis, diabetic diarrhea, neurogenic bladder, impaired cardiovascular reflexes, and impotence in men. Suggested approaches to the management of these problems are presented on page 76.

MAJOR ACUTE COMPLICATIONS

The two metabolic problems of most concern in patients with type II diabetes are nonketotic hyperglycemic hyperosmolar coma and hypoglycemia. It needs to be recognized that diabetic ketoacidosis may occur in patients with type II diabetes under severe stress.

The four major clinical features of nonketotic hyperglycemic hyperosmolar coma are
- severe hyperglycemia,
- absence of or slight ketosis,
- plasma or serum hyperosmolality, and
- profound dehydration.

Hypoglycemia can be precipitated by
- excessive insulin,
- oral hypoglycemic agents,
- decreased food intake,
- intensive exercise, and
- alcohol and other drugs.

Hypoglycemia should be suspected in a patient who presents with manifestations of altered mental and/or neurologic function as well as adrenergic responses. The diagnosis is confirmed by a plasma glucose level of less than 50 to 60 mg/dl.

If the patient is conscious, hypoglycemia should be treated by ingestion of some form of sugar by mouth. In the conscious patient, parenteral glucagon or intravenous glucose may be necessary.

ADVERSE DRUG REACTIONS

Several drugs in common use today can cause hyperglycemia or hypoglycemia (Table 28, page 79). When possible, these drugs should be avoided.

Detection and Treatment of Complications of Type II Diabetes Mellitus

INTRODUCTION

Clinicians hope that prompt identification and treatment of diabetes mellitus will be effective in averting the devastating complications of this disease. Unfortunately, even the best efforts to control hyperglycemia and to improve the patient's general health with good dietary and exercise habits are frequently unsuccessful. The patient with some type of complication is the rule rather than the exception. The number of complications that afflict patients with diabetes is extraordinary (Table 20), and a great deal has been written to enlighten the practicing physician about their importance, detection, and management.

This chapter reviews detection and treatment of the most commonly encountered major problems in patients with type II diabetes. These problems have been divided into those that are chronic and disabling and those that are acute and life threatening. In addition to chronic and acute problems, the patient with diabetes is susceptible to many adverse drug reactions, which also are discussed in this chapter because they often involve drugs that are necessary for proper care of the patient with type II diabetes (e.g., antihypertensive medications). Patient cases that illustrate proper diagnosis and treatment are presented on pages 80–83.

Pregnancy and surgery may be complicating situations in patients with diabetes mellitus. In the *Guide* they are discussed as special therapeutic problems (see Management).

There is strong, but as yet inconclusive, evidence that good metabolic control will prevent the development of long-term diabetic complications. Although attempts to normalize blood glucose should be part of the management of patients before major complications of diabetes mellitus develop, treatment goals should always balance the potential risk and benefit to the patient. The patient's age and prognosis may modify the treatment goals.

MAJOR CHRONIC COMPLICATIONS

The major chronic complications of type II diabetes mellitus include accelerated macrovascular disease, retinopathy, renal disease, foot problems, and neuropathy.

Accelerated Macrovascular Disease

In the diabetic patient, accelerated atherosclerosis involving the coronary, cerebrovascular, and peripheral vessels occurs at an earlier age and with greater frequency than it does in nondiabetic individuals. Thus, the clinician should be on the alert for signs and symptoms of accelerated atherosclerosis among diabetic patients.

Cardiovascular Complications
Studies have consistently shown that patients with diabetes mellitus have an excess of cardiovascular complications compared with nondiabetic individuals. In the United States, for example, diabetic patients are twice as prone as nondiabetic individuals to die from coronary artery disease, and the average annual incidence of cardiovascular sequelae is increased at least twofold in patients with diabetes.

Diabetes as Cardiovascular Risk Factor
As a risk factor for deaths from coronary heart disease, diabetes mellitus has a significant independent effect. The cause or causes of this excess risk are not known. However, diabetes is now considered to be one of the major macrovascular risk factors, along with hypertension, obesity, hyperlipidemia (hypercholesterolemia, hypertriglyceridemia), lack of exercise, and cigarette smoking.

Table 20. Chronic and Acute Complications Associated With Type II Diabetes Mellitus

---

MAJOR CHRONIC COMPLICATIONS

Vascular diseases

Macrovascular
- Accelerated coronary atherosclerosis
- Accelerated cerebrovascular atherosclerosis
- Accelerated peripheral vascular disease

Microvascular
- Retinopathy
- Nephropathy

Neuropathic conditions

Sensorimotor neuropathy
- Symmetrical, bilateral
  Lower extremities (most common)
  Upper extremities
- Mononeuropathy
- Neuropathic ulcer
- Diabetic amyotrophy
- Neuropathic cachexia

Autonomic neuropathy
- Gastroparesis
- Diabetic diarrhea
- Neurogenic bladder
- Impotence in men
- Impaired cardiovascular reflexes

Mixed vascular and neuropathic diseases
- Leg ulcers
- Foot ulcers

Cutaneous problems

MAJOR ACUTE COMPLICATIONS

Metabolic problems
- Nonketotic hyperosmolar hyperglycemic coma
- Hypoglycemia
- Diabetic ketoacidosis (unlikely in type II diabetes mellitus except during periods of stress such as those caused by trauma and intercurrent infection or disease)
- Lactic acidosis

Infection

Importance of Modifying Vascular Risk Factors

There are a few available prospective studies of risk factor modification in patients with type II diabetes mellitus. Even though the results of these studies are not conclusive, it is important to identify diabetic patients with high macrovascular risk profiles as early as pos-

sible and to treat them appropriately. It is important that efforts to lower plasma lipid and blood glucose levels in patients with type II diabetes be supplemented with careful control of hypertension, the latter being particularly important in terms of its benefits for reducing risks of microvascular (retinopathy and nephropathy) and macrovascular disease. Diet and exercise programs should be utilized to help patients achieve ideal weight, and cigarette smoking should be stopped.

Hypertension. There is general agreement that control of hypertension reduces the development and progression of retinopathy, nephropathy, and atherosclerosis. Treatment of hypertension in patients with diabetes should be vigorous; however, the presence of diabetes may make the patient more susceptible to some side effects of drug therapy (Table 22). For this reason, it has been difficult to achieve agreement regarding optimal drug therapy. Initial therapy may include an ACE inhibitor, a calcium channel blocker, or prazosin hydrochloride. There is controversy about the use of thiazide diuretics and beta blockers. If the blood pressure is not lowered to 140/90 mmHg or less, an alternative drug should be substituted, or a second drug should be added to the treatment program.

Lipids. In type II diabetes, an increased prevalence of lipid abnormalities contributes to accelerated atherosclerosis. Characteristically, triglyceride-rich very-low-density lipoproteins and cholesterol-rich low-density lipoproteins are elevated, whereas high-density lipoproteins are decreased. Associated obesity aggravates the lipid abnormalities. This lipid profile is the result of a combination of altered synthesis, catabolism, and clearance.

Currently, the total plasma cholesterol is used as a practical measure of lipid abnormalities. Studies indicate that adults with cholesterol levels greater than 240 mg/dl are at high risk for coronary heart disease. In most cases of type II diabetes, the elevated plasma cholesterol can be satisfactorily lowered by diet therapy. Dietary goals include (1) weight reduction if necessary, (2) a total dietary fat intake limited to 30% of total calories, (3) a saturated fat intake of no more than 10% of total calories, and (4) a daily cholesterol intake of 300 mg or less. If dietary measures fail, the addition of triglyceride- and/or cholesterol-lowering drugs is indicated.

If the patient has primarily elevated triglycerides, gemfibrozil or nicotinic acid is recommended. Nicotinic acid, previously thought to be contraindicated for patients with diabetes, is currently shown to be efficacious. If the patient primarily has elevated cholesterol, bile acid sequestrants or inhibitors of cholesterol synthesis are recommended. The recent introduction of lovastatin, an inhibitor of cholesterol synthesis, offers the clinician a new pharmacologic approach to the management of hypercholesterolemia.

Cigarette Smoking. Cigarette usage itself is associated with accelerated macrovascular disease, and the presence of diabetes in a patient who does smoke will further increase that individual's risk factors. On-going efforts should be made by the practitioner to assist the patient in discontinuing cigarette smoking, including enrollment in formal smoking cessation programs.

Diabetic Retinopathy

The importance of frequent evaluation and early detection and treatment of diabetic patients with vision problems is illustrated by the following statistics:
■ approximately 5,800 new cases of blindness related to diabetes are estimated to occur every year in the United States;
■ 50 percent of all patients with diabetes have retinopathy 10 years after diagnosis; and
■ more than 80 percent of all patients with diabetes have some form of retinopathy 15 years after diagnosis.

The following discussion is limited to diabetic retinopathy because it is often associated with serious sequelae that can be prevented if the newest diagnostic and therapeutic maneuvers are applied when indicated. The practitioner should watch for cataracts, however, because the incidence of senile cataracts among diabetic patients is greater than normal. Also, metabolic cataracts are known to be caused by sustained hyperglycemia.

Diabetic retinopathy does not cause visual symptoms until a fairly advanced stage has been reached, usually either macular edema or proliferative retinopathy. Management is more satisfactory when intervention is undertaken before visual symptoms develop. Therefore, periodic ophthalmoscopic examination by a skilled practitioner is of crucial importance.

There may well be a cause-and-effect relationship between degree of blood glucose control and subsequent development of diabetic retinopathy. Therefore, appropriate care requires close cooperation between the patient and the physician, both working toward the goal of euglycemia. At times, a specialist in diabetes may be needed, especially when a patient's blood glucose is poorly controlled.

Types of Diabetic Retinopathy

There are three types of diabetic retinopathy: (1) background diabetic retinopathy, (2) preproliferative diabetic retinopathy, and (3) proliferative diabetic retinopathy.

Background Diabetic Retinopathy (BDR). The earliest stage of BDR is recognized during ophthalmoscopic examination of the retina by the detection of microaneurysms and intraretinal "dot and blot" hemorrhages. This level of retinopathy should be expected in almost all patients with diabetes of 25 years' duration. In many cases, it does not progress.

The most common causes of visual impairment in diabetic patients with background retinopathy are macular edema and hard exudates at or near the macula. These two retinal signs often occur together. Hard exudates are usually easy to recognize with conventional direct ophthalmoscopy. Macular edema, on the other hand, is easily overlooked unless careful slit-lamp biomicroscopy is performed.

The recognition of hard exudates greater than 1 disk diameter from the center of the macula should not cause great alarm because their occurrence is rarely associated with decreased visual acuity. Macular hard exudates and edema, however, are indications for referral to an ophthalmologist who is familiar with the management of diabetic retinopathy.

Preproliferative Diabetic Retinopathy (PPDR). Certain retinal lesions represent an advanced form of background retinopathy. When a number of these lesions are found together, the risk of progression to the proliferative stage is increased. The PPDR lesions include cotton-wool spots (also referred to as soft exudates), which are ischemic infarcts in the inner retinal layers; "beading" of the retinal veins; and intraretinal microvascular abnormalities, which are dilated, tortuous retinal capillaries or, perhaps in some cases, newly formed vessels *within* the retina.

When any of these PPDR signs are found, the patient should be referred to an ophthalmologist for further evaluation. Another indication for referral is optic disk edema, which is usually benign but occasionally precedes neovascularization of the optic disk. When bilateral optic disk edema is discovered, papilledema is a possibility, and a neurologic examination is in order. A neuroophthalmologic consultation may be desirable as well.

Proliferative Diabetic Retinopathy (PDR). The final and most vision-threatening stage of diabetic retinopathy is characterized by neovascularization on the surface of the retina, sometimes extending to the posterior vitreous. The incidence of PDR among patients who have had diabetes for 15 years or more is about 30 percent. This condition is dangerous because such new vessels are prone to bleed, especially if they are stretched by contraction of the vitreous, which is a frequent occurrence in diabetes. If bleeding into the preretinal space or vitreous occurs, the patient is likely to report "floaters" or "cobwebs" in the field of vision. The patient who has a major retinal hemorrhage will experience a sudden and painless loss of vision.

The multicenter Diabetic Retinopathy Study and Early Treatment Diabetic Retinopathy Study (DRS and EDTRS) sponsored by the National Eye Institute have defined three indications for immediate referral: (1) vitreous or preretinal hemorrhage, even in the presence of normal vision; (2) neovascularization covering one-third or more of the optic disk; and (3) macular edema. The risk of severe visual loss within 2 years for patients with any high-risk characteristic is 25 to 50 percent, unless photocoagulation treatment is performed.

The proliferation of fibrous tissue that often follows PDR is a sign of remission, but its occurrence is not benign, because retinal detachment can occur as a consequence of fibrous tissue contraction.

Evaluation and Referral

The changes involved in diabetic retinopathy may be subtle and suggest that all patients with type II diabetes mellitus should have a complete visual history, visual acuity examination, and careful ophthalmoscopic examination with a dilated pupil at least once yearly. The indications for referral to an ophthalmologist are listed in Table 21.

Note that visual acuity changes are frequently related to fluctuating blood glucose levels and corresponding changes in hydration of the crystalline lens. Thus, the presenting symptom in a new patient may be a change in vision. Likewise, a patient whose blood glucose levels are suddenly decreased in response to proper treatment may experience visual acuity changes and should be forewarned as well as reassured.

Patients with visual handicaps are often classified by the ophthalmologist as follows:
■ economic visual handicap—visual acuity between 20/40 and 20/200;
■ legal blindness—visual acuity of 20/200 or less; and
■ near total or total blindness—visual acuity of less than 5/200 and inability to walk unaided.

Treatment of Retinopathy

Hypertension should be treated when present in a patient with diabetes mellitus because hypertension appears associated with increased incidence of diabetic retinopathy as well as an increased rate of progression of diabetic retinopathy. There are, however, potential complications with some antihypertensive medications (Table 22).

The ophthalmologic treatment of diabetic retinopathy depends on the stage of disease. There is no commonly accepted therapy for background retinopathy. ETDRS is evaluating this question. ETDRS demonstrated that photocoagulation slowed progressive visual loss in patients with macular exudates and edema by 50 percent.

Photocoagulation is considered the treatment of choice for patients who have proliferative retinopathy with high-risk characteristics, and it reduces the risk of severe visual loss by about 60 percent. Photocoagulation is used to stop neovascularization before recurrent hemorrhages into the vitreous cause irreparable damage. Sometimes photocoagulation is used to treat eyes with PDR before high-risk characteristics have developed. However, the risks of photocoagulation are such that usually only one eye is treated; treatment of the other eye is deferred unless high-risk characteristics develop.

When retinal detachment and massive vitreous hemorrhage occur, closed vitrectomy can be used to remove bloody vitreous and bands of fibrous tissue. During the procedure, clear fluid is infused to replace vitreous, and traction on the retina is relieved. In about 50 to 65 percent of cases, some useful sight can be restored with this procedure.

Patient Education

As the most important member of the treatment team, the patient must be fully informed about the possible visual complications of diabetes mellitus and treatment. The National Diabetes Advisory Board has suggested the following patient education principles.

■ The newly diagnosed patient should be told that diabetic retinopathy, which can cause vision loss, is a possibility and that it is important to report visual symptoms promptly.

■ The patient should be instructed regarding the possible relationship between hyperglycemia and diabetic retinopathy, with emphasis on the necessity to adhere to the prescribed treatment plan for diabetes.

■ Patients also should know that hypertension may worsen diabetic retinopathy and that its diagnosis and treatment are important.

■ The patient with diabetic retinopathy should be informed of treatment possibilities (including photocoagulation) as well as the need for referral to an ophthalmologist familiar with the management of diabetic eye problems.

■ The patient should be aware that certain exercises can aggravate proliferative retinopathy.

■ The patient who is visually impaired or blind should be made aware of and referred to vocational rehabilitation programs and other social services.

Table 21. Reasons for Referral of Patients With Type II Diabetes Mellitus to an Ophthalmologist

High-risk patients
■ Neovascularization covering more than one-third of optic disk;
■ vitreous or preretinal hemorrhage with any neovascularization, particularly on optic disk; or
■ macular edema.

Symptomatic patients
■ Blurry vision persisting for more than 1 to 2 days or not associated with a change in blood glucose;
■ sudden loss of vision in one or both eyes; or
■ black spots, cobwebs, or flashing lights in field of vision.

Asymptomatic patients
■ Yearly examinations;
■ hard exudates near macula;
■ any preproliferative or proliferative characteristics; or
■ pregnancy.

Modified from Rand LI: Retinopathy: What to look for. *Clin Diabetes* 1:14–18, 1983

Diabetic Renal Disease

The prevalence of diabetic renal disease is at least 5 to 10 percent 20 years after diagnosis in patients whose diabetes was diagnosed after the age of 30 years (presumably type II).

Clinical Presentation

The pathologic hallmarks of diabetic renal disease include nodular and, particularly, diffuse intercapillary glomerulosclerosis. These renal changes are associated with a characteristic clinical syndrome. Usually, proteinuria is the first indication of renal disease. If renal insufficiency develops, proteinuria is followed by increased levels of blood urea nitrogen and serum creatinine, and a nephrotic syndrome may develop.

Conditions That Influence Renal Function

In patients with diabetes mellitus, there are a number of conditions that either precipitate impairment of renal function or exacerbate the condition when present. These conditions include hypertension, neurogenic bladder, infection, urinary obstruction, and nephrotoxic drugs.

Table 22. Potential Complications of Antihypertensive Drugs in the Diabetic Patient

DRUG	POTENTIAL COMPLICATIONS
Diuretics	
Potassium losing	Hypokalemia
Thiazides	Hyperglycemia
Loop diuretics	Hyperlipidemia
	Impotence
Potassium sparing	Hyperkalemia
Spironolactone	Impotence
Triamterene	Gynecomastia
Vasodilators	
Hydralazine	Exacerbation of coronary
Minoxidil	heart disease
Sympathetic inhibitors	
Methyldopa	Orthostatic hypotension
Clonidine	Impotence
Guanabenz	Depression
Alpha-adrenergic blockers	
Prazosin	Orthostatic hypotension
Beta-adrenergic blockers	
Nonselective	Cardiac failure
Propranolol	Impaired insulin release with
Nadolol	hyperglycemia
Timolol	Delayed recovery from
Pindolol	hypoglycemia
Cardioselective*	Blunted symptoms of
Metoprolol	hypoglycemia
Atenolol	Hypertension associated with
	hypoglycemia
	Hyperlipidemia
Angiotensin-converting enzyme inhibitors	
Captopril	Proteinuria
Enalapril	Hyperkalemia
	Leukopenia/arganulocytosis

*Cardioselectivity may be lost with high doses.

Adapted from Christlieb AR: Treating hypertension in the patient with diabetes. *Med Clin North Am* 66:1373–88, 1982

Hypertension. A significant number of diabetic patients develop hypertension, which may precipitate the onset and further accelerate the process of renal insufficiency.

Neurogenic Bladder. Neurogenic bladder may predispose the patient to acute urinary retention or to moderate and persistent obstructive nephropathy. In either case, renal failure may be accelerated.

Infection and Urinary Obstruction. When these occur together, the risk of pyelonephritis and papillary necrosis increases, and this may result in a decline of renal function. Repetitive urethral instrumentation increases the risk of urinary tract infections. Infarction of the renal medulla and papillae can occur from ischemic necrosis, infarction, or obstruction. This patient typically presents with fever, flank pain, anuria, and accelerated loss of renal function.

Nephrotoxic Drugs. Nephrotoxic drugs, chronic analgesic abuse, and dye contrast radiographic studies have been associated with increased incidence and acceleration of renal failure in patients with diabetes. This suggests that nephrotoxic drugs should be avoided when possible and that dye contrast studies should be performed only after careful consideration of alternative procedures.

Evaluation, Treatment, and Consultation

To delay the onset and acceleration of renal disease in patients with diabetes, hypertension must be detected and, if present, treated appropriately. There are potential complications associated with the use of antihypertensive medications (Table 22), and these should be kept in mind when instituting therapy.

To monitor the onset of signs of renal damage, a urinalysis (including microscopic analysis), serum creatinine, and/or blood urea nitrogen should be done in all new patients. They also should be done yearly in all patients. The finding of proteinuria should be followed with a urine culture using the clean-voided technique. If present, infection should be treated before the significance of the proteinuria can be determined.

Consultation with a specialist is suggested if persistent proteinuria, an elevation in serum creatinine or blood urea nitrogen, or hypertension unresponsive to treatment is seen.

Patient Education

With regard to diabetic renal disease, the following patient education principles are suggested.
■ Patients should be told that diabetic renal disease is a possibility and that poor diabetes control may speed the process of renal failure.
■ Patients should be told that the detection and treatment of

hypertension is important because high blood pressure precipitates the onset of renal disease and accelerates its progression.

■ Patients should be encouraged to have their blood pressure checked regularly and to adhere to therapy when prescribed. Patients should also be encouraged to follow a no-salt-added diet and to achieve and maintain ideal body weight for the purpose of preventing or modifying the severity of hypertension.

■ The symptoms of urinary tract infection should be explained, and the patient should be instructed to report such symptoms.

■ Patients should know why treatment of hypertension and recurrent urinary tract infection is important.

■ The patient with signs of developing nephropathy should be told about the course of the disease and the options for treatment with dialysis and renal transplantation.

Diabetic Foot Problems

More than 50 percent of the nontraumatic amputations in the United States occur in individuals with diabetes, and it has been estimated that more than half of these amputations could have been prevented with proper care. Therefore, the clinician and patient who are conscientious about prevention, early detection, and prompt treatment of diabetic foot problems can have significant impact on this problem.

Cause of Diabetic Foot Problems
Foot lesions in individuals with diabetes mellitus are the result of peripheral neuropathy, peripheral vascular disease, superimposed infection, or, most often, a combination of these complications. Usually, foot lesions are found in feet that are insensitive, deformed, and ischemic. Such feet are susceptible to trauma, which may lead to ulceration, infection, and gangrene.

In most diabetic patients with foot lesions, the primary pathophysiologic event is the development of an insensitive foot. Hyperglycemia is almost invariably associated with mild defects in nerve conduction, and the feet are highly susceptible to becoming insensitive. If treated early, mild nerve conduction defects are reversible. Loss of foot sensation is often, but not always, accompanied by decreased vibratory sense and loss of ankle jerk reflexes. Sometimes diabetic neuropathy is accompanied and worsened by other types of neuropathy, most commonly alcoholic peripheral neuropathy.

In addition to insensitivity, neuropathy may ultimately lead to a deformed foot secondary to tendon shortening (contractures), which leads to decreased mobility of the toes, abnormality in weight bearing, and development of classic "hammertoe" deformities. The combination of foot insensitivity and foot deformities that allow undue stress on small areas of the foot promotes the development of foot ulcers. Neuropathy also causes decreased sweating and dry skin. If left untreated, cracked and thickened skin will eventually lead to ulcerations.

Neuropathic ulcers in the diabetic patient often go undetected because they are usually painless. When pain occurs, the prognosis is usually poor because it generally means infection with bone involvement.

The sudden development of a painful distal foot lesion, usually secondary to trauma, often signifies underlying peripheral vascular disease, which is usually associated with findings of decreased pulses, dependent rubor, and pallor on elevation. The extent of the vascular disease and its potential for treatment by surgical intervention can be determined by Doppler noninvasive techniques and arteriography. Unfortunately, surgical intervention is not always effective because individuals with diabetes may have diffuse vascular disease.

Infection is a frequent complication of both vascular and neuropathic ulcers. Studies indicate that these infections are usually mixed and that gram-positive organisms predominate.

Prevention of Foot Problems
The prevention of foot problems in a person with diabetes requires proper foot care by the patient as well as early detection and prompt treatment of lesions by the physician. Help from special health-care professionals (podiatrist, orthopedist, vascular surgeon, and experts in shoe fitting) is frequently needed.

Table 23. Risk Factors for Diabetic Foot Problems

- Age greater than 40
- Cigarette smoking
- Diabetes mellitus of more than 10 years' duration
- Decreased peripheral pulses or sensation
- Anatomic deformities (bunions, hammertoes, prominent metatarsal heads)
- History of foot ulcers, amputations

Physician Responsibility. The first step in prevention is to educate all patients (see below) and to identify those who need a special evaluation frequently because of risk factors for foot problems (Table 23). During the evaluation, the examiner should determine whether the patient has experienced foot problems or intermittent claudication since the last visit. The physician also should conduct a thorough examination of both feet, looking for the signs and symptoms of impending foot problems (Table 24), which include foot deformities and ulcers. The clinician should also check the pulses (dorsalis pedis, popliteal, tibial, and femoral), search for bruits, and determine vibratory sensation in the toes and feet.

Patient Responsibility. The patient who has been given necessary information and proper instruction should assume major responsibility for prevention of foot problems. The patient (or family member, in the case of a patient who is impaired by morbid obesity, severe retinopathy, or blindness) should be given instruction on how to file calluses, to cut toenails straight across, and to inspect the feet daily for cuts, abrasions, and corns. The patient and family should know the importance of regular washing with warm water and mild soap followed by thorough drying. They should be instructed on the use of moistening agents such as lanolin, and the need to avoid strong chemicals such as epsom salt or iodine. The potential hazards of heat, cold, new shoes, constricting or mended socks, and going barefoot should be emphasized.

Treatment of Foot Problems

Minor noninfected wounds can be treated with nonirritating antiseptic solution, daily dressing changes, and foot rest. However, more serious problems such as foot deformities, infected lesions, and ulcers are best handled in consultation with specialists in diabetic foot care.

Neuropathic Conditions

The diabetic neuropathies are among the most common and perplexing complications of diabetes mellitus. A complete dissertation on the peripheral and visceral (autonomic) neuropathies is beyond the scope of the *Guide*. Instead, a few important points about diagnosis and treatment of commonly encountered neuropathic problems are discussed.

Sensorimotor Neuropathy

The peripheral neuropathies include the symmetrical bilateral neuropathies of the upper and lower extremities, various specific mononeuropathies, neuropathic ulcer (described above), diabetic amyotrophy, and neuropathic cachexia.

Symmetrical Bilateral Neuropathy. This problem may occur in the upper extremities but is more common in the lower. It may be nearly asymptomatic (poorer prognosis) or very painful, particularly at night. The absence of deep reflexes, especially ankle jerks, is a valuable objective finding. The painful forms may subside spontaneously in 6 months but may persist for years.

In general, there is little evidence that any drug therapy is useful in diabetic neuropathy. The B vitamins have been used extensively but have not been proven effective. There are reports that treatment with phenytoin, carbamazepine, or antidepressant medication such as amitriptyline may be helpful in some patients. Aldose reductase inhibitors are being evaluated as therapeutic agents, but their use is still in the experimental stage. Aspirin or propoxyphene should be prescribed as necessary for pain.

Mononeuropathy. The mononeuropathies are asymmetrical, abrupt in onset, and usually painful. Extraocular muscle motor paralysis, particularly that innervated by the third and sixth nerves, is the most noticeable of the mononeuropathies. Spontaneous recovery in about 3 months is usual.

Table 24. Warning Symptoms and Signs of Diabetic Foot Problems

	SYMPTOMS	SIGNS
Vascular	■ Cold feet ■ Intermittent claudication involving calf or foot ■ Pain at rest, especially nocturnal, relieved by dependency	■ Absent pedal, popliteal, or femoral pulses ■ Femoral bruits ■ Dependent rubor, plantar pallor on elevation ■ Prolonged capillary filling time (>3–4 seconds) ■ Decreased skin temperature
Neurologic	■ Sensory: burning, tingling, or crawling sensations; pain and hypersensitivity; cold feet ■ Motor: weakness (drop foot) ■ Autonomic: diminished sweating	■ Sensory: deficits (vibratory and proprioceptive, then pain and temperature perception), hyperesthesia ■ Motor: diminished to absent deep tendon reflexes (Achilles then patellar), weakness ■ Autonomic: diminished to absent sweating
Musculoskeletal	■ Gradual change in foot shape ■ Sudden painless change in foot shape, with swelling, without history of trauma	■ Cavus feet with claw toes ■ Drop foot ■ "Rocker-bottom" foot (Charcot's joint) ■ Neuropathic arthropathy
Dermatologic	■ Exquisitely painful or painless wounds ■ Slow-healing or nonhealing wounds, or necrosis ■ Skin color changes (cyanosis, redness) ■ Chronic scaling, itching, or dry feet ■ Recurrent infections (e.g., paronychia, athlete's foot)	**Skin** ■ Abnormal dryness ■ Chronic tinea infections ■ Keratotic lesions with or without hemorrhage (plantar or digital) ■ Trophic ulcer **Hair** ■ Diminished to absent **Nails** ■ Trophic changes ■ Onychomycosis ■ Subungual ulceration or abscess ■ Ingrown nails with paronychia

From Scardina RJ: Diabetic foot problems: assessment and prevention. *Clin Diabetes* 1:1–7, 1983

Diabetic Amyotrophy. Diabetic amyotrophy is characterized by severe pain, wasting of the proximal muscles (pelvic girdle and thigh), and minimal to absent sensory involvement. It is usually asymmetrical and more common in men. Prominent features include quadriceps involvement, atrophy of thigh muscles, and absent patellar tendon reflexes. Complete healing usually occurs in several months to a year.

Neuropathic Cachexia. This syndrome is characterized by exquisite pain and profound weight loss. It usually occurs in men who are in their 60s. Anorexia, impotence, and peripheral symmetrical, bilateral neuropathy are frequent findings. Spontaneous recovery occurs in about 12 months.

Autonomic Neuropathy

The autonomic neuropathies, which usually occur in concert with peripheral neuropathy, include gastroparesis, diabetic diarrhea, neurogenic bladder, impaired cardiovascular reflexes, and impotence in men.

Table 25. Differential Diagnosis of Impotence in Diabetic Men

TYPE	LIBIDO	ERECTION LOSS	NOCTURNAL AND MORNING ERECTIONS	SPECIAL PARTNER ERECTIONS	MASTURBATION ABILITY
Diabetic	Normal	Gradual	Absent	Absent	Partial/total
Psychological	Decreased	Abrupt	Present	Present	Impaired

Kozak GP: Impotence in diabetic males. In *World Book of Diabetes in Practice 1982*. Krall LP, Alberti KGMM, Eds. Amsterdam, Excerpta Medica, 1982, p. 108–12

Gastroparesis. The patient with gastroparesis may experience nausea, vomiting, and abdominal discomfort in response to delayed emptying or retention of gastric contents. Metoclopramide, in doses of 10 milligrams three to four times a day, is often helpful. On occasion, larger doses are required.

Diabetic Diarrhea. Frequent passage of loose stools, particularly after meals and at night, marks the acute phase of this condition. Diabetic diarrhea tends to be intermittent. Some patients respond to treatment with a broad-spectrum antibiotic such as tetracycline. However, other treatments, such as diphenoxylate (Lomotil) and metoclopramide, have been shown to be quite effective.

Neurogenic Bladder. Neurogenic bladder is characterized by a gradual loss of ability to void. The demonstration of cystometric abnormalities and residual urine are necessary for diagnosis. Surgical intervention may be required if the patient does not respond to conservative medical measures, because chronic urinary retention may lead to infection followed by hydropyelonephritis, renal failure, and death.

Impaired Cardiovascular Reflexes. Orthostatic hypotension and increased heart rates may occur when autonomic neuropathy affects the cardiovascular reflexes. Patients with orthostatic hypotension may find relief with use of 9-α-fluorohydrocortisone, compression stockings, an abdominal binder, or, if necessary, an Air Force antigravity suit. If 9-α-fluorohydrocortisone is prescribed, the initial dose should be as low as 0.1 milligram, and increases up to 1.0 milligram should be made gradually. The drug should be used with particular caution in patients with cardiac disease, because it is associated with salt and water retention and, thus, can precipitate congestive heart failure. Clonidine, a central alpha$_2$-receptor blocking agent, has been used recently to treat this condition.

Impotence in Men. Impotence is a frequent occurrence in men with diabetes and usually manifests itself by lack of firm, sustained erection. In most cases, libido and ejaculatory function are not affected. Table 25 presents some of the distinguishing characteristics of diabetic and psychogenic impotence. The measurement of nocturnal penile tumescence (NPT) is sometimes used to determine whether the patient's erections during sleep are normal, borderline, or abnormally diminished for age. When psychogenic and endocrine causes of impotence have been ruled out, the implantation of a semirigid or inflatable penile prosthesis allows the patient to resume sexual intercourse. Intrapenile injections of vasodilating substances (papaverine and phentolamine) have shown promise as an alternative treatment.

MAJOR ACUTE COMPLICATIONS

The major acute complications of diabetes mellitus include metabolic problems and infection.

Metabolic Problems

The two metabolic problems of most concern in patients with type II diabetes are nonketotic hyperglycemic hyperosmolar coma and hypoglycemia.

Table 26. Factors Associated With Nonketotic Hyperglycemic Hyperosmolar Coma

THERAPEUTIC AGENTS	THERAPEUTIC PROCEDURES	CHRONIC DISEASE	ACUTE SITUATIONS
Glucocorticoids	Peritoneal dialysis	Renal disease	Infection
Diuretics	Hemodialysis Hyperosmolar alimentation Surgical stress	Heart disease Hypertension Old stroke Alcoholism	Diabetic gangrene Urinary tract infection Septicemia Extensive burns
Diphenylhydantoin		Psychiatric Loss of thirst	Gastrointestinal hemorrhage
Beta-adrenergic blocking agents			Cerebrovascular accident Myocardial infarction Pancreatitis
Diazoxide			
L-Asparaginase			
Immunosuppressive agents			
Chlorpromazine			

Garcia de los Rios M: Nonketotic hyperosmolar coma. In *World Book of Diabetes Practice 1982*. Krall LP, Alberti KGMM, Eds. Amsterdam, Excerpta Medica, 1982, p. 96–99; and Podolsky S: Hyperosmolar nonketotic coma. In *Diabetes Mellitus*. Vol. V. Rifkin H, Raskin P, Eds. Bowie, MD, Brady, 1981, chapt. 22

Nonketotic Hyperglycemic Hyperosmolar Coma

Of all diabetic comas, nonketotic hyperglycemic hyperosmolar coma is the most common in older patients with type II diabetes mellitus. When this condition occurs, it can be life threatening. This metabolic problem sometimes occurs spontaneously in people with undiagnosed diabetes mellitus and in known diabetic patients after long periods of uncontrolled hyperglycemia.

Precipitating Causes. Almost always there is a precipitating factor (Table 26). Precipitating events include the use of potential hyperglycemia-inducing agents and procedures as well as other acute and chronic diseases and conditions (particularly infection).

Clinical Presentation. There are four major clinical features of nonketotic hyperglycemic hyperosmolar coma:
■ severe hyperglycemia (blood glucose >600 mg/dl and generally between 1,000 and 2,000 mg/dl);
■ absence of or slight ketosis;

■ plasma or serum hyperosmolality (>340 mosM of water); and
■ profound dehydration.

Typically, the patient develops altered sensorium (coma or confusion), physical signs of severe dehydration, shallow respirations, excessive thirst, and the absence of an odor of acetone on the breath.

Treatment. The precipitating event should be determined and corrected as soon as possible while life-saving measures are immediately employed. Dehydration, hyperglycemia, and the hyperosmolar condition should be corrected with use of appropriate fluids, insulin, and potassium.

Hypoglycemia

This metabolic problem occurs in both type I and type II diabetic patients.

Precipitating Causes. Usually hypoglycemia is precipitated by excessive insulin, oral hypoglycemic agents, decreased food intake, excessive exercise, and alcohol and other drugs.

Table 27. Common Infections in Patients With Diabetes Mellitus

TYPE OF INFECTION	COMMENT
Cutaneous **Furunculosis** **Carbuncles**	For reasons not particularly clear, patients with diabetes mellitus may be prone to recurrent furunculosis and carbuncles. Unless vascular insufficiency is present, warm compresses may be used for treatment.
Vulvovaginitis (less frequently, scrotal infections)	*Candida* skin infection commonly occurs in warm, moist areas, particularly in the region of the genitalia (also on the inner thighs and under the breasts). This is particularly common in type II diabetic patients who are overweight or who have been taking antibiotics. These infections can cause extreme discomfort to the patient and result in breakdown of skin, which may allow entry of more virulent organisms. Good diabetic control and local supportive antifungal treatment usually will resolve the problem.
Cellulitis, alone or in combination with lower extremity vascular ulcers	To prevent the spread of infection to bone and the necessity of amputation, treatment of infected ulcers and surrounding cellulitis must be aggressive. Antibiotics effective against bacteria recovered from the site (both aerobes and anaerobes should be expected), as well as surgical debridement and drainage, should be used.
Urinary tract	Asymptomatic bacteriuria occurs in up to 20 percent of patients with diabetes mellitus; some suggest that it be treated. Certainly a patient with neurogenic bladder is susceptible to urinary tract infection and sepsis. Treatment is mandatory in patients with pyelonephritis. Patients with serious urinary tract infections should be hospitalized, the offending pathogens identified, and appropriate susceptibility tests performed.
Pulmonary	Pneumonia is the most frequent infection in patients with diabetes. Most often the causative organism is *Streptococcus pneumoniae,* but gram-negative organisms are found in a large number of cases. Prompt evaluation with a chest film, sputum smear (gram and acid-fast strains), and sputum culture are necessary. Transtracheal aspiration may be necessary if the patient is not producing sputum. Initial therapy should be based on the sputum gram strain.
Ear	Malignant external otitis is most often seen in elderly patients with chronically draining ear and sudden onset of severe pain. *Pseudomonas aeruginosa* is the usual pathogenic organism. This condition is fatal in about 50 percent of cases. Immediate treatment should include appropriate antibiotic therapy and surgical debridement when indicated.

From Rabinowitz, SG: Infection in the diabetic patient. In *Diabetes Mellitus.* Vol. V. Rifkin H, Raskin P, Eds. Bowie, MD, Brady, 1981, chapt. 24; and Casey JI: Host defense and infections in diabetes mellitus. In *Diabetes Mellitus: Therapy and Practice.* 3rd ed. Ellenberg M, Rifkin H, Eds. New Hyde Park, NY, Medical Examination Publishing, 1983, chapt. 32

Clinical Presentation. Hypoglycemia should be suspected in a patient who presents with symptoms indicative of altered mental and/or neurologic function (changes in sensorium and behavior, coma, or seizure), as well as adrenergic responses (tachycardia, palpitations, increased sweating, and hunger). The diagnosis is confirmed if a plasma glucose level of less than 50 to 60 mg/dl is found when the patient is symptomatic.

Treatment. The objective of treatment is to restore the plasma glucose level to normal. When the patient remains conscious, ingestion of some form of sugar by mouth (e.g., fruit juice, sugar cubes, glucose tablets, or a solution equivalent to 5–20 grams of carbohydrate) is usually followed by rapid relief of symptoms. Parenteral glucagon may be used to treat severe hypoglycemic reactions. In the unconscious pa-

Table 28. Drugs That Alter Sulfonylurea Action

DRUGS THAT ENHANCE HYPOGLYCEMIC ACTIVITY
Effect sulfonylurea pharmacokinetics
Displacement from albumin binding site
- Clofibrate
- Halofenate
- Phenylbutazone, oxyphenylbutazone, and sulfinpyrazone
- Salicylates
- Some sulfonamides

Prolongs half-life by interfering with metabolism
- Bihydroxycoumarin
- Chloramphenicol
- Monoamine oxidase inhibitors
- Sulfaphenazole
- Pyrazolone derivatives (e.g., phenylbutazone)

Decreased urinary excretion
- Allopuriol
- Probenecid
- Pyrazolone derivatives (e.g., phenylbutazone)
- Salicylates
- Some sulfonamides

Have their own intrinsic hypoglycemic activity
- Alcohol
- Salicylates
- Guanethidine
- Monoamine oxidase inhibitors
- Beta blockers

DRUGS THAT ANTAGONIZE SULFONYLUREA ACTION AND CAUSE HYPERGLYCEMIA
Effect sulfonylurea pharmacokinetics
Shorten half-life by increasing metabolism
- Chronic alcohol use
- Rifampin

Have own intrinsic hyperglycemic activity
- Acetazolamide
- Beta blockers
- Diazoxide
- Diuretics (e.g., thiazides, furosemide)
- Epinephrine
- Estrogens
- Glucagon
- Glucocorticoids
- Indomethacin
- Isoniazid
- Nicotinic acid
- Phenytoin
- L-Thyroxine

tient, intravenous injection of glucose should be given.

Infection

The rapid diagnosis and treatment of infection in a patient with diabetes mellitus is absolutely necessary because infection is a leading cause of metabolic abnormalities leading to diabetic coma. The more common infections seen in patients with diabetes mellitus and some critical comments about them are presented in Table 27.

ADVERSE DRUG REACTIONS

There are several drugs in common use today that adversely affect the diabetic patient because they may cause hyper- or hypoglycemia. These drugs should be prescribed with caution (Table 28).

PATIENT CASES

The following cases illustrate the most important points about diagnosis and management of the major complications of type II diabetes mellitus.

Case 1: The 51-Year-Old Executive Secretary

A.W., a 51-year-old executive secretary with type II diabetes mellitus of 15 years' duration treated with diet alone (although she had a course of treatment with tolbutamide for 6 years until 5 years ago), presents with a 3 to 4 month history of progressive exertional dyspnea and easy fatigability. She reports no chest pain, except for an occasional episode of nonspecific chest discomfort after protracted sexual intercourse. She has not experienced nocturnal dyspnea, orthopnea, or peripheral edema. She reports a history of smoking one pack of cigarettes per day for 35 years. Her family has no history of diabetes or cardiac disease.

Physical examination reveals a blood pressure of 138/85, a pulse of 88 beats per minute, and mild background diabetic retinopathy. The cardiovascular examination shows a normal-sized heart without gallops or murmurs and good peripheral pulses without bruits.

Laboratory studies reveal a fasting plasma glucose level of 181 mg/dl, serum cholesterol of 295 mg/dl, triglycerides of 160 mg/dl, glycosylated hemoglobin of 10.1 percent, and serum creatinine of 1.1 mg/dl. ECG and chest X-ray are unremarkable.

Because of the progressive nature of symptoms, an exercise radionuclide flow study (MUGA scan) is performed. It reveals a decreased ejection fraction after exercise and some anterior wall dyskinesia. To further evaluate this finding, an exercise thallium study is performed and shows a cold area demonstrable only with exercise.

Coronary arteriography is recommended and performed. During the procedure, the patient is well hydrated, and a minimal amount of contrast dye is employed. Proximal lesions are identified in all three coronary vessels, with no distal lesions and good runoff.

The patient was referred for coronary artery bypass surgery. Six months after triple-bypass coronary artery surgery, the patient was symptom-free and stable.

Discussion Points

■ Coronary artery disease is the leading cause of death in patients with type II diabetes, who have a two- to fivefold increased risk of coronary disease compared with the general population. The presentation is often atypical chest pain. Myocardial infarctions in diabetic patients can be "silent" and occur without pain.

■ Diabetic patients often have involvement of more than one coronary artery. Contrary to popular myth, the lesions are often proximal and amenable to coronary bypass surgery. The 5-year survival rates for diabetic and nondiabetic patients with equivalent degrees of coronary disease are nearly equal.

■ Because of the risk of contrast-dye-induced acute renal failure, coronary arteriography should be performed under conditions of good hydration with a minimal amount of contrast material.

■ Smoking markedly potentiates the risk of coronary artery disease, and patients should be admonished to cease smoking.

■ The hallmark of diabetic hyperlipidemia is hypertriglyceridemia, which usually is proportional to the degree of hyperglycemia and responsiveness to glucose control.

■ In patients with type II diabetes, hypercholesterolemia is common, usually mild, generally due to an increase of low-density lipid cholesterol, and usually responsive to good dietary management, including weight control, control of hyperglycemia, and reduction of cholesterol and saturated fat intake.

Case 2: The 48-Year-Old Accountant

C.B., a 48-year-old Black accountant with type II diabetes of 12 years' duration treated with diet and tolazamide, presents to you for general medical care, having just moved into your community. His history is unremarkable except for some increased fatigability. Physical examination reveals a blood pressure of 185/105, pulse of 84 beats per minute, and fundi with some arteriolar narrowing, a few microaneurysms, and hard exudates. The patient has mild cardiomegaly with a prominent S_4 but no murmurs. The remainder of the examination is within normal limits.

Laboratory studies show a fasting plasma glucose level of 205 mg/dl, glycosylated hemoglobin of 9.9 percent, urinalysis with trace proteinuria, and a serum creatinine of 1.9 mg/dl. The ECG reveals left ventricular hypertrophy, and the chest X-ray shows an enlargement of the cardiac silhouette.

Repeat blood pressure measurements on three other occasions are 190/105, 180/100, and 183/105. There is no postural drop.

Treatment was initiated with atenolol. In response to progressively increasing doses, the blood pressure fell to 155/95 and the pulse to 55 beats per minute. Prazosin was added, and the blood pressure fell to 145/90. With the addition of clonidine, the blood pressure was satisfactorily maintained in the range of 125–135/80–85. With this treatment, the patient felt well.

Discussion Points

■ Coexisting hypertension is of major concern in patients with type II diabetes mellitus because it increases the risks of atherosclerosis, renal disease, and proliferative diabetic retinopathy. It should be vigorously controlled, particularly in the presence of renal insufficiency, because adequate blood pressure control slows the rate of progression of nephropathy.

■ All major studies of intervention for the treatment of hypertension have used "real world" casual blood pressure measurements. Such measurements should be the focus of attention, particularly if the diastolic blood pressure exceeds 95 mmHg or if there is coexisting cardiomegaly.

■ The objective of blood pressure control should be to maintain the blood pressure as near normal as possible (i.e., 120–135/80–85) without postural hypotension.

■ Diuretics are usually used first in the treatment of hypertension. However, diuretic agents impair endogenous insulin secretion and, thus, may exacerbate hyperglycemia in some patients. Diuretic use also may be associated with hemoconcentration, fluid and electrolyte imbalance, hyperuricemia, hyperlipidemia, and impotence.

■ Antihypertensive agents that may be preferred in diabetic patients include a cardioselective beta-blocking drug (a cardioselective beta blocker such as atenolol does not impair the epinephrine response to hypoglycemia unless used in large doses), a direct vasodilator (e.g., prazosin), and a centrally acting drug (e.g., clonidine). To promote patient compliance, the simplest possible dosage schedules should be used. ACE inhibitors and calcium channel antagonists may have a useful role in the treatment of hypertension in type II diabetes.

■ Renal insufficiency in patients with type II diabetes (especially among Black individuals) is a concern. Renal involvement generally begins 10 to 12 years after diagnosis of diabetes. Annual urinalysis should be performed to detect renal involvement. If proteinuria is found, a serum creatinine or creatinine clearance should be obtained.

Case 3: The 56-Year-Old Lawyer

P.L., a 56-year-old lawyer with type II diabetes of 8 years' duration treated with diet and insulin, presents in your office for routine follow-up. When he undresses for his physical examination, he leaves his shoes and socks on. You ask him to remove them, and he replies that it is unnecessary to do so because his feet are fine. You insist. Examination of his left foot reveals a small (1.5 centimeters in diameter) painless ulcer on the plantar surface over the first metatarsal head.

Physical examination also reveals absent Achilles reflexes, decreased vibration over the great toes and malleoli, and generalized sensory loss over the feet, with a stocking distribution. Peripheral pulses are intact, and the feet are normal in temperature.

Culture of the wound reveals mixed

flora, and an X-ray of the foot is unremarkable.

The wound is cleaned, and the patient is placed on bed rest.

Discussion Points

■ The feet should be examined frequently, especially in patients older than 40, those with diabetes of more than 10 years' duration, and those with a history of neuropathy, peripheral vascular disease, or foot problems. Such evaluation should include seeking a history of foot problems, paresthesias, or intermittent claudication; inspection of the feet, toes, and toe webs for ulcers, calluses, cleanliness, deformities, and fit of shoes; palpation of peripheral pulses (dorsalis pedis, posterior tibial); and determination of sensation (especially vibration) and intactness of ankle reflexes.

■ The patient should be taught proper foot care, including regular daily inspection of feet, filing calluses, cutting toenails straight across, not walking barefoot, washing feet regularly, using lanolin to prevent drying, breaking in new shoes slowly, avoiding heat or self-medication, and promptly seeking medical care for all foot lesions.

■ A warm, insensitive foot (i.e., neuropathic and pain insensitive) is at greater risk than a cool ischemic foot that feels pain.

■ Once an ulcer appears in an insensitive foot, there should be absolutely no weight on the lesion. Antibiotics and debridement should be used as necessary.

■ Peripheral vasculature can be evaluated by a Doppler stethoscope, determining the systolic pressure index (ratio of ankle pressure to brachial pressure). Values below 0.9 signify the presence of vascular insufficiency.

■ Patients with recently healed ulcers or with insensitive feet should try to decrease amount of walking, speed of walking, and size of steps.

Case 4: The 46-Year-Old Registered Nurse

H.M., a 46-year-old registered nurse with type II diabetes of 9 years' duration treated with diet and insulin therapy, presents for routine follow-up examination.

Physical examination includes a funduscopic examination through dilated pupils. This reveals multiple microaneurysms, "dot and blot" hemorrhages, some hard exudates, and a few soft exudates. The patient is referred to an ophthalmologist.

Visual acuity is 20/20 bilaterally. The optic media are clear. Ophthalmoscopy confirms the presence of microaneurysms, dot and blot hemorrhages, and both hard and soft exudates. In addition, a few areas of venous dilation and some intraretinal microvascular abnormalities are noted. No maculopathy or neovascularization is seen. Photographs of the fundi confirm the above.

A follow-up ophthalmologic appointment is arranged for 6 months later.

Discussion Points

■ Funduscopic examination should always be carried out through dilated pupils by an examiner experienced in the diagnosis and classification of diabetic retinopathy. A primary care physician must decide whether to develop the requisite expertise or to refer patients to an ophthalmologist for such examinations.

■ Funduscopic examination should be done yearly. The patient should be referred for regular follow-up by an ophthalmologist experienced in the evaluation and treatment of diabetic retinopathy when retinopathy is detected or suspected, when the patient presents with ocular symptoms, or when difficulty is experienced in performing the funduscopic examination.

■ Most patients with diabetic retinopathy, including proliferative retinopathy, experience no visual symptoms.

■ Hypertension in patients with diabetes is associated with an increased incidence and rate of progression of diabetic retinopathy; therefore, hypertension should be rigorously sought and vigorously treated in patients with diabetes mellitus.

■ Certain characteristics of diabetic retinopathy indicate a high risk for loss of vision, which can be lessened by treatment with photocoagulation.

These high-risk characteristics are (1) new vessels and preretinal or vitreous hemorrhage; (2) new vessels on or within 1 disk diameter of the optic disk $\geq \frac{1}{4}$ to $\frac{1}{3}$ the disk area in extent, even in the absence of preretinal or vitreous hemorrhage; and (3) macular edema.

■ Diabetes is a leading cause of new blindness among adults in the United States. Nevertheless, only a minority of diabetic patients will develop the type of retinopathy that threatens vision. The risk of blindness can be substantially reduced with careful and regular evaluations for early detection and with appropriate use of current therapeutic tools.

Case 5: The 58-Year-Old Contractor

N.C., a 58-year-old contractor with type II diabetes of 19 years' duration treated with diet and tolazamide, presents for his annual physical examination. During review of systems, he reports progressive erectile failure of approximately 1 year duration. He says the problem began with inability to maintain erections, followed by inability to achieve vaginal penetration, and most recently inability to achieve any erection. Libido persists, but the patient is quite discouraged about his erectile incompetence. He reports no morning erections, does not use any medications except tolazamide, and rarely consumes alcohol.

Physical examination is unremarkable except for decreased vibratory sensation in the lower extremities at the great toes and absent Achilles reflexes. SMA-12 is unremarkable except for a plasma glucose level of 174 mg/dl.

Urologic evaluation demonstrates normal genitalia but absent bulbocavernous and bulbosphincteric reflexes. Penile plethysmography reveals a normal penile blood pressure. NPT studies show absence of tumescence activity consistent with organic impotence. Serum testosterone and prolactin are normal. The urologist requests psychological consultation, including psychological testing. Results are normal.

The patient was referred for surgical implantation of an inflatable penile prosthesis. Both he and his wife are satisfied with the results.

Discussion Points

■ Psychogenic factors are the major cause of impotence in both diabetic and nondiabetic men. Even when organic factors are present, many men have ambiguous impotence due to a combination of psychogenic and organic factors.

■ Neuropathic impotence in diabetic men is usually associated with coexisting peripheral neuropathy. There is a higher incidence of neuropathic bladder changes in impotent diabetic patients than in nonimpotent diabetic men. The bulbocavernous and bulbosphincteric reflexes are often absent in men with neuropathic impotence.

■ Neuropathic impotence is generally manifested by progressive erectile failure. Ejaculatory capacity usually is not affected.

■ The most effective test for differentiating organic and psychogenic impotence is the NPT test.

■ The implantation of a penile prosthetic device is a highly satisfactory and acceptable method for the treatment of erectile failure.

BIBLIOGRAPHY

Casey JI: Host defense and infections in diabetes mellitus. In *Diabetes Mellitus: Theory and Practice*. 3rd ed. Ellenberg M, Rifkin H, Eds. New Hyde Park, NY, Medical Examination Publishing, 1983, chapt. 32

Dyck PJ, Thomas PK, Asbury AK: *Diabetic Neuropathy*. Philadelphia, PA, Saunders, 1987

Early Treatment of Diabetic Retinopathy Study Research Group: Photocoagulation of diabetic macular edema: early treatment diabetic retinopathy study report no. 1. *Arch Ophthalmol* 103:1796–806, 1985

Garcia de los Rios M: Nonketotic hyperosmolar coma. In *World Book of Diabetes Practice 1982*. Krall LP, Alberti KGMM, Eds. Amsterdam, Excerpta Medica, 1982, p. 96–99

Kaplan NM, Rosenstock J, Raskin P: A differing view of treatment of hypertension in patients with diabetes mellitus. *Arch Intern Med* 147:1160–62, 1987

Keen H, Jarrett J (Eds.); *Complications of Diabetes.* London, Arnold, 1982

Klein R, Klein BEF, Moss SE, et al: The Wisconsin epidemiologic study of diabetic retinopathy. III. Prevalence and risk of diabetic retinopathy when age of diagnosis is 30 or more years. *Arch Ophthalmol* 102:527–32, 1984

Klein R, Moss SE, Klein BEK: New management concepts for timely diagnosis of diabetic retinopathy treatable by photocoagulation. *Diabetes Care* 10:633–38, 1987

Levin ME, O'Neal W (Eds.): *The Diabetic Foot.* 3rd ed. St. Louis, MO, Mosby, 1983

Marble A, Krall LP, Bradley RF (Eds.): In *Joslin's Diabetes Mellitus.* 12th ed. Philadelphia, PA, Lea & Febiger, 1985

National Diabetes Advisory Board: *The Prevention and Treatment of Five Complications of Diabetes: A Guide for Primary Care Practitioners.* Washington, DC, U.S. Department of Health and Human Services, 1983, NIH publ. no. 83-8392

National Diabetes Advisory Board: *The Treatment and Control of Diabetes: A National Plan to Reduce Mortality and Morbidity.* Washington, DC, Department of Health and Human Services, 1980, NIH publ. no. 81-2284, p. 25

Rabinowitz SG: Infection in the diabetic patient. In *Diabetes Mellitus.* Vol. V. Rifkin H, Raskin P, Eds. Bowie, MD, Brady, 1981, chapt. 24

Rand LI: Retinopathy: what to look for. *Clin Diabetes* 1:14–18, 1983

Rosenthal J, Raskin P: Early diabetic nephropathy: assessment and potential therapeutic interventions. *Diabetes Care* 9:525–45, 1986

Scardina RJ: Diabetic foot problems: assessment and prevention. *Clin Diabetes* 1:1–7, 1983

Seltzer HS: Adverse drug interactions of clinical importance to diabetes. In *Diabetes Mellitus.* Vol. V. Rifkin H, Raskin P, Eds. Bowie, MD, Brady, 1981, chapt. 40

The Diabetic Retinopathy Study Research Group: Photocoagulation treatment of proliferative diabetes: clinical application of diabetic retinopathy, (DRS) study findings. *Ophthalmology* 88:583–600, 1981

The Working Group on Hypertension in Diabetes: Statement on hypertension in diabetes mellitus: final report. *Arch Intern Med* 147:830–42, 1987

Index,
ADA Information

Index

ADA Information

Affiliates
Clinical Education Program
Professional Membership

Index

E

Exercise, 32–36
  benefits, 32–33
    adjunct to diet, 33
    cardiovascular, 33
    improvement in insulin sensitivity/
      glucose tolerance, 32–33
    other, 33
  energy expenditure with exercises,
    36
  guidelines for prescription, 34–35
    appropriate exercise program,
      34–35
    detailed medical evaluation, 34
    individualization, 34–35
    instructions to patient, 35
    special concerns, 35
      active proliferative retinopathy,
        35
      hypertension, 35
      hypoglycemia, 35
      insensitive feet, 35
  indications and contraindications, 34
  risks, 34–35

F

Fat. *See* Diet therapy
Fiber. *See* Diet therapy
Foot problems, 73–74, 75
  cause, 73
  incidence and risk, 74
  prevention, 73–74
    patient responsibility, 74
    physician responsibility, 74
  risk factors, 74
  treatment, 74
  warning signs and symptoms, 75
Fructose. *See* Diet therapy

G

Gastroparesis. *See* Neuropathic
conditions
Gestational diabetes mellitus (GDM).
See Glucose intolerance
Glipizide (Glucatrol), 38, 39
Glucatrol. *See* Glipizide
Glucose intolerance, 3–11
  diagnosis, 6–9, 10
    diagnostic tests, indications and
      criteria, 7–9, 10
    oral glucose tolerance test, 8, 9
    screening, indications and criteria,
      6–7, 8
  distinguishing characteristics of
    clinical classes, 3–6
    diabetes mellitus, 3–5, 6
    gestational diabetes mellitus, 4,
      5–6

    impaired glucose tolerance, 4, 5
    distinguishing characteristics of
      statistical risk classes, 4, 6
    evaluation and classification, 4, 6,
      9–11
Glucose tolerance test. *See* Tests/
Testing
Glyburide (Diabeta, Micronase), 38,
39
**Glycosylated hemoglobin
concentration.** *See* Assessment of
therapy

H

Home blood glucose monitoring. *See*
Assessment of therapy
Hyperinsulinemia. *See* Pathogenesis of
non-insulin-dependent (type II)
diabetes mellitus
Hypertension, 29, 35, 68, 70, 72–73,
80, 81
  dietary therapy, 29
  importance of treatment, 68, 70,
    72–73, 80, 81
    macrovascular disease, 68
    patient case histories, 80, 81
    renal disease, 72–73
    retinopathy, 70
  potential complications of
    antihypertensive medication, 72
  precautions in exercise, 35
Hypoglycemia, 34–35, 38, 39, 77–78,
79
  acute metabolic problems, 77–78
    clinical presentation, 78
    precipitating causes, 77
    treatment, 78
  drugs that enhance hypoglycemic
    activity, 79
  exercise-induced, 34–35
  side effect of sulfonylurea therapy,
    38, 39

I

Impaired glucose tolerance (IGT). *See*
Glucose intolerance
Impotence in men. *See* Neuropathic
conditions
Infection, 78, 79
  common infections in diabetic
    patients, 78
  importance of treatment, 78, 79
**Insulin-dependent (type I) diabetes
mellitus,** 3–4
  evaluation and classification, 9–12
Insulin resistance. *See* Pathogenesis of
non-insulin-dependent (type II)
diabetes mellitus
Insulin secretion. *See* Pathogenesis of

O

choice of agent, 39
complications, 39
contraindications, 37
drug failures, 39–40
drugs that alter sulfonylurea action, 79
drugs that enhance hypoglycemic activity, 79
mechanism of action, 25, 38
oral agent plus insulin, 44–45
patients likely to respond, 37
Orinase. *See* Tolbutamide

P

Pathogenesis of non-insulin-dependent (type II) diabetes mellitus, **15–19**
glucose-stimulated insulin response, 15–16
physiologic consequences of, 16
insulin resistance, 16–17
mechanisms of, 17
sites of, 16–17
insulin secretion, 15
fasting insulin concentration, 15
pathogenetic sequences, 17–19
primary beta-cell defect, 17–19
primary cellular defect, 19
Patient attitudes and concerns, 57–63
emotional responses to diabetes, 57–58
significant issues, 58–61
complications, 61
frequent visits to physician, 60–61
physical activity (exercise), 59–60
self-monitoring of urine and blood, 60
weight reduction, 59
Patient case histories, 78–82
Patient education, 25, 26, 32, 33, 35, 37, 44, 46, 51, 57–63, 71, 72–73, 74
behavior modification techniques for weight reduction, 61
importance in management, 26, 32, 33, 35, 37, 44, 46, 59–60, 61, 71, 72–73, 74
diet therapy, 26, 32, 59
exercise, 33, 35, 59–60
pharmacologic intervention, 37, 44
pregnancy, 46
prevention of complications, 61, 71, 72–73, 74
key to successful therapy, 25
relationship to compliance, 58, 61–63
role in self-monitoring, 51, 60
Pharmacologic intervention. *See* Drug therapy
Physical activity. *See* Exercise
Plasma glucose determinations. *See*

Assessment of treatment; Tests/ Testing
Pregnancy, 8–9, 10, 45–46
diagnosis of gestational diabetes, 8–9, 10
management, 45–46
Preproliferative diabetic retinopathy (PPDR). *See* Retinopathy
Proliferative diabetic retinopathy (PDR). *See* Retinopathy
Protein. *See* Diet therapy

R

Renal disease, 71–73
clinical presentation, 71
conditions that influence renal function, 71–72
hypertension, 72
infection, 72
nephrotoxic drugs, 72
neurogenic bladder, 72
urinary obstruction, 72
evaluation, 72
incidence, 71
management, 72
consultation with specialist, 72
treatment of hypertension, 71
patient education, 72–73
Retinopathy, 69–71, 72
classification of visual handicap, 70
evaluation, 70
incidence and risks, 69
indications for referral to ophthalmologist, 70
management, 70–71
photocoagulation, 70–71
treatment of hypertension, 71, 72
vitrectomy, 71
patient education, 71
types of retinopathy, 69–70
background diabetic retinopathy, 69
preproliferative diabetic retinopathy, 69–70
proliferative diabetic retinopathy, 70

S

Saccharin. *See* Diet therapy
Screening tests. *See* Tests/Testing
Self-monitoring of blood glucose. *See* Assessment of treatment
Sensorimotor neuropathy. *See* Neuropathic conditions
Sulfonylurea drugs. *See* Oral hypoglycemic agents
Surgery. *See* Management of non-insulin-dependent (type II) diabetes mellitus

Affiliates

American Diabetes Association
ALABAMA AFFILIATE, INC.
3 Office Park Circle
Suite 115
Birmingham, AL 35223
(205) 870-5172; (205) 870-5173;
1-800-824-7891

American Diabetes Association
ALASKA AFFILIATE, INC.
201 E. 3rd Avenue
Suite 301
Anchorage, AK 99501
(907) 276-3607

American Diabetes Association
ARIZONA AFFILIATE, INC.
7337 North 19th Avenue
Room 404
Phoenix, AZ 85021
(602) 995-1515

American Diabetes Association
ARKANSAS AFFILIATE, INC.
Tanglewood Shopping Center
7509 Cantrell Road
Suite 227
Little Rock, AR 72207
(501) 666-6345

American Diabetes Association
CALIFORNIA AFFILIATE, INC.
2031 Howe Avenue
Suite 250
Sacramento, CA 95825
(916) 925-0199

American Diabetes Association
COLORADO AFFILIATE, INC.
2450 South Downing Street
Denver, CO 80210
(303) 778-7556

American Diabetes Association
CONNECTICUT AFFILIATE,
   INC.
P.O. Box 10160 (mailing address)
40 South Street
West Hartford, CT 06110
(203) 249-4232; (800) 842-6323

American Diabetes Association
DELAWARE AFFILIATE, INC.
2713 Lancaster Avenue
Wilmington, DE 19805
(302) 656-0030

American Diabetes Association
WASHINGTON, D.C., AREA
   AFFILIATE, INC.
1819 H Street, N.W.
Suite 1200
Washington, DC 20006
(202) 331-8303

American Diabetes Association
FLORIDA AFFILIATE, INC.
P.O. Box 19745 (mailing address)
Orlando, FL 32814
3101 Maguire Blvd., Suite 288
Orlando, FL 32803
(305) 894-6664

American Diabetes Association
GEORGIA AFFILIATE, INC.
3783 Presidential Parkway
Suite 102
Atlanta, GA 30340
(404) 454-8401

American Diabetes Association
HAWAII AFFILIATE, INC.
510 South Beretania Street
Honolulu, HI 96813
(808) 521-5677

American Diabetes Association
IDAHO AFFILIATE, INC.
1528 Vista
Boise, ID 83705
(208) 342-2774

American Diabetes Association
DOWNSTATE ILLINOIS
   AFFILIATE, INC.
965 North Water Street
Decatur, IL 62523
(217) 422-8228

American Diabetes Association
NORTHERN ILLINOIS
   AFFILIATE, INC.
6 North Michigan Avenue
Suite 1202
Chicago, IL 60602
(312) 346-1805

American Diabetes Association
INDIANA AFFILIATE, INC.
222 South Downey Avenue
Suite 320
Indianapolis, IN 46219
(317) 352-9226

American Diabetes Association
IOWA AFFILIATE, INC.
888 Tenth Street
Marion, IA 52302
(319) 373-0530

American Diabetes Association
KANSAS AFFILIATE, INC.
3210 East Douglas
Wichita, KS 67208
(316) 684-6091

American Diabetes Association
KENTUCKY AFFILIATE, INC.
McClure Building, #513
P.O. Box 345 (mailing address)
306 West Main, #513
Frankfort, KY 40602
(502) 223-2971

American Diabetes Association
LOUISIANA AFFILIATE, INC.
9420 Lindale Avenue
Suite B
Baton Rouge, LA 70815
(504) 927-7732

American Diabetes Association
MAINE AFFILIATE, INC.
P.O. Box 2208 (mailing address)
c/o S. Parish Congregational Church
9 Church Street
Augusta, ME 04330
(207) 623-2232

American Diabetes Association
MARYLAND AFFILIATE, INC.
3701 Old Court Road
Suite 19
Baltimore, MD 21208
(301) 486-5516

American Diabetes Association
MASSACHUSETTS AFFILIATE,
 INC.
190 North Main Street
Natick, MA 01760
(617) 655-6900

American Diabetes Association
MICHIGAN AFFILIATE, INC.
The Clausen Building North Unit
23100 Providence Drive
Suite 475
Southfield, MI 48075
(313) 552-0480

American Diabetes Association
MINNESOTA AFFILIATE, INC.
3005 Ottawa Avenue, South
Minneapolis, MN 55416
(612) 920-6796

American Diabetes Association
MISSISSIPPI AFFILIATE, INC.
10 Lakeland Circle
Jackson, MS 39216
(601) 981-9511

American Diabetes Association
MISSOURI AFFILIATE, INC.
P.O. Box 1674 (mailing address)
213 Adams Street
Jefferson City, MO 65102
(314) 636-5552

American Diabetes Association
MONTANA AFFILIATE, INC.
P.O. Box 2411
Great Falls, MT 59403 (mailing
 address)
600 Central Plaza, Suite 304
Great Falls, MT 59401
(406) 761-0908

American Diabetes Association
NEBRASKA AFFILIATE, INC.
2730 South 114th Street
Omaha, NE 68144
(402) 333-5556

American Diabetes Association
NEVADA AFFILIATE, INC.
4550 East Charleston Boulevard
Las Vegas, NV 89104
(702) 459-7099

American Diabetes Association
NEW HAMPSHIRE AFFILIATE,
 INC.
P.O. Box 595 (mailing address)
Manchester, NH 03105
104 Middle Street
Manchester, NH 03101
(603) 627-9579

American Diabetes Association
NEW JERSEY AFFILIATE, INC.
P.O. Box 6423 (mailing address)
312 North Adamsville Road
Bridgewater, NJ 08807
(201) 725-7878

American Diabetes Association
NEW MEXICO AFFILIATE, INC.
525 San Pedro, N.E.
Suite 101
Albuquerque, NM 87108
(505) 266-5716

American Diabetes Association
NEW YORK DOWNSTATE
   AFFILIATE, INC.
505 8th Avenue
New York, NY 10018
(212) 947-9707

American Diabetes Association
NEW YORK UPSTATE
   AFFILIATE, INC.
P.O. Box 1037 (mailing address)
Syracuse, NY 13201
115 East Jefferson Street
Syracuse, NY 13202
(315) 472-9111

American Diabetes Association
NORTH CAROLINA AFFILIATE,
   INC.
2315-A Sunset Avenue
Rocky Mount, NC 27801
(919) 937-4121

American Diabetes Association
NORTH DAKOTA AFFILIATE,
   INC.
P.O. Box 234
Grand Forks, ND 58206-0234
   (mailing address)
101 North 3rd St.
Suite 502
Grand Forks, ND 58201
(701) 746-4427

American Diabetes Association
OHIO AFFILIATE, INC.
705L Lakeview Plaza Court
Columbus, OH 43085
(614) 436-1917

American Diabetes Association
OKLAHOMA AFFILIATE, INC.
Warren Professional Building
6465 South Yale Avenue
Suite 423
Tulsa, OK 74136
(918) 492-3839 or 1 (800) 722-5448

American Diabetes Association
OREGON AFFILIATE, INC.
3607 S.W. Corbett Street
Portland, OR 97201
(503) 228-0849

American Diabetes Association
GREATER PHILADELPHIA
   AFFILIATE, INC.
21 South Fifth Street
The Bourse
Suite 570
Philadelphia, PA 19106
(215) 627-7718

American Diabetes Association
MID-PENNSYLVANIA
   AFFILIATE, INC.
2045 Westgate Drive
Suite B-1
Bethlehem, PA 18017
(215) 867-6660

American Diabetes Association
WESTERN PENNSYLVANIA
   AFFILIATE, INC.
4617 Winthrop Street
Pittsburgh, PA 15213
(412) 682-3392

American Diabetes Association
RHODE ISLAND AFFILIATE,
   INC.
4 Fallon Avenue
Providence, RI 02908
(401) 331-0099

American Diabetes Association
SOUTH CAROLINA AFFILIATE,
   INC.
P.O. Box 50782 (mailing address)
2838 Devine Street
Columbia, SC 29250
(803) 799-4246

American Diabetes Association
SOUTH DAKOTA AFFILIATE,
   INC.
P.O. Box 659 (mailing address)
Sioux Falls, SD 57101
1524 West 20th Street
Sioux Falls, SD 57105
(605) 335-7670

American Diabetes Association
TENNESSEE AFFILIATE, INC.
1701 21st Avenue, South
Room 403
Nashville, TN 37212
(615) 298-9919

American Diabetes Association
TEXAS AFFILIATE, INC.
8140 North Mopac
Building 1
Suite 130
Austin, TX 78759
(512) 343-6981

American Diabetes Association
UTAH AFFILIATE, INC.
643 East 400 South
Salt Lake City, UT 84102
(801) 363-3024

American Diabetes Association
VERMONT AFFILIATE, INC.
217 Church Street
Burlington, VT 05401
(802) 862-3882

American Diabetes Association
VIRGINIA AFFILIATE, INC.
404 8th Street, N.E.
Suite C
Charlottesville, VA 22901
(804) 293-4953

American Diabetes Association
WASHINGTON AFFILIATE, INC.
3201 Fremont Avenue North
Seattle, WA 98103
(206) 632-4576; 1-800-628-8808

American Diabetes Association
WEST VIRGINIA AFFILIATE,
  INC.
Professional Building
1036 Quarrier Street
Room 404
Charleston, WV 25301
(304) 346-6418; 1-800-642-3055

American Diabetes Association
WISCONSIN AFFILIATE, INC.
10721 W. Capitol Drive
Milwaukee, WI 53222
(414) 464-9395

American Diabetes Association
WYOMING AFFILIATE, INC.
2908 Kelly Drive
Cheyenne, WY 82001
(307) 638-3578; (307) 237-2325

Clinical Education Program (CEP)
from the American Diabetes Association

ADDITIONAL MATERIALS TO ENHANCE THE PHYSICIAN'S GUIDE . . .

Principles of Good Care in the Management of Type II Diabetes Mellitus

The accompanying slide set to the *Physician's Guide*. Available in English or Spanish (please specify on order), plus script (in English only). 116 slides. 1984. #034
Nonmember: $49.90; Member: $39.90

Lecture Notes

A workbook to complement the above slide set. 32 pages. Softcover. 1984. #035
Nonmember: $3.75; Member: $3.00

Forty Commonly Asked Questions About Type II Diabetes (NIDDM)

This booklet was developed from hundreds of questions and answers collected at the CEP Conference. 36 pages. Softcover. 1984. #036
Nonmember: $3.75; Member: $3.00

The Diagnosis and Treatment of Diabetes Mellitus Type II

Video or film. Six diabetes experts discuss type II diabetes.
Video: 3/4" #031 or VHS #032 or Beta #033
Nonmember: $49.90; Member: $39.90
16mm Film: #030
Nonmember: $249.00; Member: $199.00

NEW
Physician's Guide to Insulin-Dependent (Type I) Diabetes: Diagnosis and Treatment

This handbook is an essential reference manual for the health-care professional, covering all problems—from diagnosis to complications of IDDM. 1988. #038
Nonmember: $20.00; Member: $16.00

NEW
Clinical Diabetes Reviews, Volume I

This new book covers the most important topics in the treatment of diabetes. *CDR* is a compilation of articles (1983–1987) taken from *Clinical Diabetes* and *Diabetes Care*. 200 pages.
Softcover. 1987. #408
Nonmember: $19.95; Member: $15.95

Goals for Diabetes Education

This book covers all the goals and objectives of effective diabetes education in an easy-to-use checklist format. 48 pages.
Softcover. 1987. #201
Nonmember: $6.00; Member: $4.80

ADA Publications Order Form

Name _____

Address _____

City _____ State _____ Zip _____

☐ Check here to receive a FREE *ADA Publications Catalog*.
☐ I am an ADA member. My member number is

HJ02

_____
(appears on your *Diabetes Forecast* label)

Item No.	Title	No. of Copies		Price		Total
_____	_____	_____	×	$_____	=	$_____
_____	_____	_____	×	$_____	=	$_____
_____	_____	_____	×	$_____	=	$_____
_____	_____	_____	×	$_____	=	$_____
				Total Amount Enclosed		$_____

Please make your check payable to the American Diabetes Association. Send your completed order form and payment to: American Diabetes Association, 1660 Duke St., Alexandria, VA 22314, Attn: Order Department. Allow 6–8 weeks for delivery. All prices include shipping and handling charges.

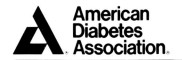
American Diabetes Association.

Application for Professional Membership
(please print)

Name_____

Title_____ Organization/Institution_____

Address_____

City_____ State_____ Zip_____

Phone (_____) _____   Is this your ☐ Home or ☐ Office?

Education: Degree_____   Specialty_____ Date Earned _____

Degree_____   Specialty_____ Date Earned _____

PROFESSIONAL SECTION MEMBERSHIP DIRECTORY INFORMATION

Please check your specialty or specialties (up to 3) for your Directory listing:

☐ Administration (AD)   ☐ Epidemiology (EP)   ☐ Nutrition (NU)   ☐ Pharmacy (PM)
☐ Anatomy (AN)   ☐ Endocrinology (EN)   ☐ Obstetrics/Gynecology (OG)   ☐ Physiology (PY)
☐ Anesthesiology (AE)   ☐ Family Practice (FP)   ☐ Ophthalmology (OP)   ☐ Podiatry (PO)
☐ Biology (BI)   ☐ General Practice (GP)   ☐ Optometry (OT)   ☐ Psychiatry (PS)
☐ Biochemistry (BC)   ☐ Geriatrics (GE)   ☐ Orthopedics (OR)   ☐ Psychology (PC)
☐ Cardiology (CA)   ☐ Internal Medicine (IM)   ☐ Osteopathy (OS)   ☐ Public Health (PH)
☐ Dentistry (DO)   ☐ Immunology (IU)   ☐ Pathology (PT)   ☐ Research (RE)
☐ Dermatology (DE)   ☐ Metabolism (ME)   ☐ Pediatric Diabetes (PD)   ☐ Social Worker (SW)
☐ Diabetes (DM)   ☐ Nephrology (NE)   ☐ Pediatric Endocrinology (PN)   ☐ Surgery (SU)
☐ Dietetics (DN)   ☐ Neurology (NR)   ☐ Pediatrics (PE)   ☐ Urology (UR)
☐ Education (ED)   ☐ Nursing (NS)   ☐ Pharmacology (PA)   ☐ Other _____

Please check one of the following locations:

☐ Academic (1)   ☐ Hospital (3)   ☐ Public Health (5)   ☐ Other (7)
☐ Clinic (2)   ☐ Office Based (4)   ☐ Research (6)   ☐ Retired (8)

FREE COUNCIL MEMBERSHIP

Please check your selection. FULL PROFESSIONAL MEMBERS receive *two free* Councils Memberships. All other members receive *one free* council membership. Additional Council Memberships are available for $25 each.

New! ☐ Council on Complications (TT)   New! ☐ Council on Education (SS)   New! ☐ Council on Exercise (XX)
☐ Council on Diabetes in Pregnancy (BB)   New! ☐ Council on Foot Care (RR)   ☐ Council on Health Care (DD)
☐ Council on Diabetes in Youth (EE)   ☐ Council on Epidemiology   ☐ Council on Nutritional
and Statistics (CC)   Sciences and Metabolism (AA)

MEMBERSHIP CATEGORY/DUES INFORMATION

Please check appropriate membership category.

	Full Membership*	Research Focus	Clinical Focus	Associate
Regular	☐ $150.00	☐ $ 90.00	☐ $ 90.00	☐ $50.00
Student**	☐ $ 75.00	☐ $ 45.00	☐ $ 45.00	☐ $25.00
International***	☐ $225.00	☐ $140.00	☐ $140.00	☐ $80.00

*   M.D.'s must select this category.
** If you've received your first professional degree, diploma, or certificate during the preceding 5 years, be sure to list your
     degree information in the space provided on the membership form.
***Includes *all* members living outside the U.S. and Canada. All publications will be expedited within 18 days or less.

☐ I am enclosing $_____ for membership.
☐ I am enclosing $_____ for _____ additional Council(s).
TOTAL AMOUNT ENCLOSED $_____

The portion of the membership dues that is set aside for publications is as follows: DIABETES $50.00 (in-training members $25.00); DIABETES CARE $35.00 (in-training members $17.50); DIABETES FORECAST $14.00 (in-training members $7.00); DIABETES SPECTRUM $20.00 (in-training members $10.00).

If you need specific information not available here, use our toll-free number 1-800-232-3472. In Alaska, Hawaii and Virginia please call 703-549-1500.

Please allow 5-7 weeks for the processing of your order.

Please send completed application with your dues payment to: American Diabetes Association, Professional Section Membership, 1660 Duke Street, Alexandria, VA 22314. Attn: Pat McKay.

HGII

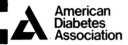

American Diabetes Association

The ADA Professional Section ... New Membership Categories And Benefits Designed Specifically For You.

New Membership Categories!

In order to better serve your professional interests, the ADA now offers you the choice from among four membership categories:

FULL PROFESSIONAL MEMBERSHIP—Includes all physicians. Also includes all other health-care professionals who wish to receive the full range of professional section benefits. (Physicians must join this category). Annual Dues: $150.00

RESEARCH FOCUS MEMBERSHIP—Includes Ph.D's, researchers, and scientists studying diabetes. Annual Dues: $90.00

CLINICAL FOCUS MEMBERSHIP—Includes nurses, dietitians, pharmacists, diabetes educators, and other health-care professionals who devote at least 50% of their time to patients with diabetes. Annual Dues: $90.00

ASSOCIATE PROFESSIONAL MEMBERSHIP—Includes same professionals as Clinical Focus Membership, who devote less than 50% of their time to diabetic patients. Annual Dues: $50.00.

If you have received your first professional degree within the last five years you are eligible to become a Member-In-Training. This qualifies you for dues at half-price. Just be sure to list your degree information in the space provided on the membership form.

Publications

NEW!
- **DIABETES SPECTRUM**
- **DIABETES**
- **DIABETES CARE**
- **CLINICAL DIABETES**
- **DIABETES FORECAST**
- **DIABETES '88**
- **PROFESSIONAL SECTION REPORT**

ADA publications offer continuing education for professionals. You're as close to the latest research and up-to-date information on treatment and care as you are to your mailbox. (see box for publications offered for each membership category).

FREE Council Membership

- Your opportunity to learn and serve on your choice from nine ADA Special Interest Councils. Select your council(s) from the list on the other side.

Professional Membership Directory

Your link to a valuable network of more than 8,000 diabetes experts.

PROFESSIONAL MEMBERSHIP CATEGORIES AT A GLANCE

BENEFITS	Full Professional Membership	Research Focus	Clinical Focus	Associate Professional
Diabetes	•	•		
Diabetes Care	•		•	
Diabetes Spectrum	•		•	•
Clinical Diabetes	•	•	•	
Diabetes Forecast	•		•	•
Diabetes '88	•	•	•	•
Professional Section Report	•		•	•
Free Councils	2	1	1	1
Annual Membership Directory	•		•	•
Discounts on Educational Programs	•	•	•	•
Grants & Awards	•	•	•	•
Voting Rights	•		•	
Membership in local ADA Affiliate	•	•	•	
Discount on Registration to BRS "Colleague"	•	•	•	•

Grants and Awards

- Members of the ADA Professional Section are eligible to receive grants to support diabetes research. In addition, annual awards are presented to physicians, educators, and researchers to honor outstanding performances.

Discounts on Educational Programs

- Save on registrations for ADA's Scientific Sessions and the Postgraduate Course.

Voting Rights and Privileges

- Your national ADA membership also entitles you to membership at the local affiliate level where you can vote and actively participate in shaping the future of ADA. Through your participation in locally sponsored professional and patient education programs, you can help the ADA improve the well-being of all people with diabetes. Through the products and services we provide our professional members, ADA is helping you and your colleagues to get closer and closer to the cure. Join ADA today.

On-Line Library Access

- Discount of $25 when you subscribe to *BRS Colleague*, the computerized medical library. Members can now access *Colleague* via their personal computers to review selected ADA publications plus a comprehensive library of non-ADA journals and books.

American Diabetes Association, Inc.

Publisher
CAROLINE STEVENS

Director of Professional Publications
BEVERLY BRITTAN COOK

Managing Editor
ORIT LOWY

Revision Editor
ARLENE KARIDIS

Design Coordinator
STEPHEN J. CHICHERIO